ACUTE PHASE PROTEINS

Edited by **Sabina Janciauskiene**

Acute Phase Proteins
http://dx.doi.org/10.5772/46063
Edited by Sabina Janciauskiene

Contributors

Manuel Bicho, Alda Pereira Da Silva, Maria Clara Bicho, Rui Medeiros, Sabina Janciauskiene, Csilla Tothova, Oskar Nagy, Herbert Seidel, Gabriel Kovac, Mao, Cheng-Yu Chen, Paul Kenneth Witting, Masaki Otagiri, Kazuaki Taguchi, Koji Nishi, Victor Tuan Giam Chuang, Toru Maruyama, Simon Davidson

Published by InTech

Janeza Trdine 9, 51000 Rijeka, Croatia

Publishing Process Manager Sandra Bakic
Technical Editor InTech DTP team
Cover InTech Design team

Additional hard copies can be obtained from orders@intechopen.com

Acute Phase Proteins , Edited by Sabina Janciauskiene
p. cm.
ISBN 978-953-51-1185-6

For EU product safety concerns:
IN TECH d.o.o., Prolaz Marije Krucifikse Kozulić 3, 51000 Rijeka, Croatia,
info@intechopen.com or visit our website at intechopen.com.

Meet the editor

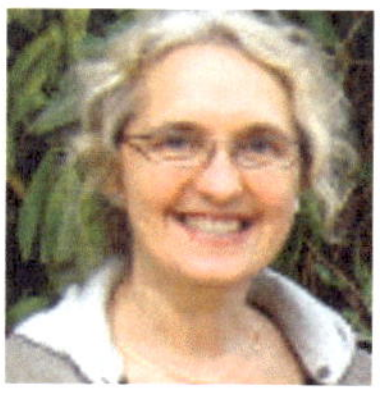

Prof. Dr. Sabina Janciauskiene was born in 1960 in Sweden. Since 1992, overall objective of her research is to investigate the mechanisms controlling inflammation, with particular emphasis on the multiple roles played by serine protease inhibitors (serpins) like: alpha1-antitrypsin and alpha1-antichymotrypsin. Dr. Janciauskiene`s group was among the first to propose that serpin misfolding can also occur due to post-translational modifications of serpin molecule, such as oxidation, nitration, interaction with other molecules and cleavage. Dr. Janciauskiene is a member of the German Lung Research Center and European Respiratory Society. She is a receiver of several prices Teggers Stipendium, King`s Gustaf V & Queen`s Victoria Award and International ALTA "B Laurell Award, for new insights in Alpha1-antitrypsin deficiency field, among others. Dr. Janciauskiene made substantial contributions through publications, book chapters, external oral/poster presentations, organizing conferences, contribution to the diagnostic test research and development, and active participation within the Leonardo Da Vinci educational program in Europe, and collaboration with Alpha1-Antitrypsin deficiency patient organizations in Sweden, Germany, and England.

Contents

Preface

Acute phase proteins (APPs) are a large group of proteins synthesized by the liver cells and released into the bloodstream in response to a variety of stressors as part of the acute phase of the inflammatory reaction. Proteins with a transient increase in synthesis and plasma concentration are called positive, whereas proteins whose synthesis decreases are referred to as negative APPs. The synthesis of the APP is thought to be mainly regulated by inflammatory cytokines, such as interleukin-6, interleukin-1 and tumor necrosis factor.

APPs functioning as protease inhibitors, enzymes, transport proteins, coagulation proteins, and modulators of the host's immune response, and play a role in the restoration of homeostasis after injury or infection. APPs act in a time, concentration and molecular conformation-dependent manner on a variety of cells involved in early and late stages of inflammation. APPs can directly contribute to the enhancement and/or the suppression of inflammation at different points in its evolution. The administration of specific APPs has been shown to switch the pro-inflammatory to the anti-inflammatory pathways necessary for the resolution of inflammation in vitro and in vivo. Nevertheless, the biological function of most APPs has not been totally elucidated. It is also not clear what functional advantages may arise from the rapid changes in the blood profile of APPs as a group.

Thus, the magnitude and rapidity of the changes in the specific profile of APPs, together with their short half-life, suggest a particularly important role for these proteins in the establishment of host defense. The functional activities of specific APPs and their quantification during the course of acute and chronic inflammation are discussed in this book.

Prof. Dr. Sabina Janciauskiene
Department of Respiratory Medicine,
Hannover Medical School,
Hannover, Germany

Chapter 1

Immunoregulatory Properties of Acute Phase Proteins — Specific Focus on α1-Antitrypsin

S. Janciauskiene, S. Wrenger and T. Welte

Additional information is available at the end of the chapter

http://dx.doi.org/10.5772/56393

1. Introduction

Activation of innate immune cells in response to various insults is a part of the host defence. However, if uncontrolled, this inflammatory response induces persistent hyper-expression of pro-inflammatory mediators and tissue damage. Tight control of pro-inflammatory pathways is therefore critical for immune homeostasis and host survival.

A complex network of activating and regulatory pathways controls innate immune responses; the hepatic acute-phase response is one of the crucial contributors to this regulation. For example, in response to infection or tissue injury within few hours the pattern of protein synthesis by the liver is drastically altered, i.e. increased expression of the so called positive acute phase proteins (APPs) like C-reactive protein (CRP), alpha1-antitrypsin (AAT) or alpha1-acid glycoprotein (AGP) and decreased expression of transthyretin, retinol binding protein, cortisol binding globulin, transferrin and albumin, which represent the group of negative APPs. This production of APPs in hepatocytes is controlled by a variety of cytokines released during inflammation whereas leading regulators are IL-1- and IL-6-type cytokines having additive, inhibitory, or synergistic effects. For instance, IL-1β is shown to almost completely abrogate IL-6-induced production of α2-macroglobulin and α1-antichymotrypsin but, in contrast, to enhance production of CRP and serum amyloid A. No doubt, this specific regulation of AAPs expression plays a critical role in the regulation of the host innate immune responses.

2. Alpha1-antitrypsin and the acute phase response

AAT, also referred to as alpha$_1$-proteinase inhibitor or SERPINA1, is the most abundant serine protease inhibitor in human blood. AAT consists of a single polypeptide chain of 394 amino acid residues containing one free cysteine residue and three asparagines-linked carbohydrate side-chains. AAT is mainly produced by liver cells but can also be synthesized by blood monocytes, macrophages, pulmonary alveolar cells, and by intestinal and corneal epithelium (Geboes et al., 1982; Perlmutter et al., 1985; Ray et al., 1982). In terms of tissue expression AAT has been demonstrated in the kidney, stomach, small intestine, pancreas, spleen, thymus, adrenal glands, ovaries and testes. De novo synthesis of AAT has also been demonstrated in human cancer cell lines. These observations indicate that AAT transcription is relatively widespread. In fact, tissue-specific promoter activity for AAT has been reported in the liver, the major source of AAT, and alternative promotors for other tissues that express the protein (Kalsheker et al., 2002; Tuder et al., 2010). Interestingly, AAT expression also shows some degree of substrate and/or auto-regulation: upon exposure to neutrophil and pancreatic elastases, either alone or as a complex of AAT, enhanced synthesis of AAT was observed (Perlmutter et al., 1988).

The normal daily rate of synthesis of AAT is approximately 34 mg/kg body weight and the protein is cleared with a half-life of 3 to 5 days. This results in high plasma concentrations ranging from 0.9 to 2 mg/ml when measured by nephelometry. In addition to high circulating levels in blood, AAT is also present in saliva, tears, milk, semen, urine and bile (Berman et al., 1973; Chowanadisai & Lonnerdal, 2002; Huang, 2004; Janciauskiene et al., 1996; Poortmans & Jeanloz, 1968). The distribution of the protein in the tissues is not uniform. For example, in the epithelial lining fluid of the lower respiratory tract its concentration is approximately 10% of plasma levels (Janciauskiene, 2001).

As an acute-phase reactant, circulating AAT levels increase rapidly (3 to 4 fold) in response to inflammation or infection. The concentration of AAT in plasma also increases during oral contraceptive therapy and pregnancy. During an inflammatory response, tissue concentrations of AAT may increase as much as 11-fold as a result of local synthesis by resident or invading inflammatory cells (Boskovic & Twining, 1997). Blood monocytes and alveolar macrophages can contribute to tissue AAT levels in response to inflammatory cytokines (IL-6, IL-1 and TNFα) and endotoxins (Knoell et al., 1998; Perlmutter & Punsal, 1988). Recent data demonstrate that AAT expression by alpha and delta cells of human islets (Bosco et al., 2005) and intestinal epithelial cells (Faust et al., 2001) is also enhanced by pro-inflammatory cytokines. AAT synthesis by corneal epithelium, on the other hand, appears to be under the influence of retinol, IL-2, fibroblast growth factor-2, and insulin-like growth factor-I (Boskovic & Twining, 1997; Boskovic & Twining, 1998). Oncostatin M, a member of the IL-6 family was shown to induce AAT production by human bronchial epithelial cells. This effect of oncostatin M was in turn modulated by TGF-β and IFN-γ at both the protein and mRNA level. IFN-γ decreased oncostatin M-induced AAT production whilst TGF-β induced a significant and synergistic up-regulation of AAT that was not observed in a hepatocyte cell line (Boutten et al., 1998). Study by Shin and coworkers (Shin et al., 2011) have demonstrated that nasal lavage fluids from the patients with allergic rhinitis contains AAT and that the levels of nasal AAT markedly increase in response to allergenic stimulation. This response seems to be closely associated with the activation of eosinophils induced by allergen-specific IgA. In allergen-induced nasal inflammation, AAT might be a byproduct of the activated inflammatory cells, and is thus implicated in the allergic immune response (Shin et al., 2011).

According to recent studies, activated neutrophils and eosinophils can store and secrete AAT, which plays a role in protection of tissues at local inflammation sites (Johansson et al., 2001; Paakko et al., 1996). Furthermore, Clemmensen and coworkers found that the mRNA for AAT increases during maturity of the myeloid cell precursors and is even higher in blood neutrophils. This in itself is quite remarkable as blood neutrophils are generally considered transcriptionally inactive, but it is even more striking that the transcriptional activity of the AAT gene increases further when neutrophils migrate into tissues (Clemmensen et al., 2011). Moreover, circulating AAT produced by liver cells can enter granulocytes and is stored in the secretory vesicles (Borregaard et al., 1992).

3. Protective anti-inflammatory, immunomodulatory and antimicrobial effects of alpha1-antitrypsin

Findings from different experimental models provide clear evidence that AAT expresses broad anti-inflammatory and immunoregulatory activities (Figure 1). AAT has been reported to inhibit neutrophil superoxide production, adhesion, and chemotaxis, to enhance insulin-induced mitogenesis in cell lines and to induce IL-1 receptor antagonist, a negative regulator to IL-1 signalling, in blood monocytes and neutrophils (Tuder et al., 2010). Findings that AAT enhances the synthesis of transferrin receptor and ferritin revealed a role of AAT in iron metabolism (Graziadei et al., 1997). In murine models, exogenous human AAT protects islet cell allografts from rejection and increase survival in an allogeneic marrow transplantation models. In other models AAT therapy protects against TNF-α / endotoxin induced lethality, cigarette smoke induced emphysema and inflammation and even suppressed bacterial proliferation during infections ((Lewis, 2012), review). Furthermore, human AAT given to mice during renal ischemia–reperfusion (I/R) injury lessens tissue injury and attenuated organ dysfunction (Daemen et al., 2000).

These beneficial impacts of AAT are incompletely understood, although exscinding knowledge suggests that AAT promotes a switch from pro-inflammatory to anti-inflammatory pathways necessary for the resolution of inflammation.

AAT has long been thought of as a main inhibitor of neutrophil elastase, proteinase 3, and other serine proteases released from activated human neutrophils during an inflammatory response. In fact, the rate of formation of the AAT/neutrophil elastase inhibitory complex is one of the fastest known for serpins (6.5x 10^7 M^{-1} s^{-1}) (Gettins, 2002). The structure of AAT consists of three β-sheets (A, B, C) and 9 α-helices (A-I). The inhibitory active conformation of AAT like for other serine protease inhibitors represents a metastable state, characterized by an exposed reactive center loop that acts as bait for the target enzyme (Stocks et al., 2012). Cleavage of the scissile bond in the loop results in a large conformational change in which the reactive site loop migrates and is inserted into the pre-existing β-sheet A forming a very stable complex between the inhibitor and the protease. This reaction results in a rapid and irreversible inactivation of both AAT and its target protease.

As an inhibitor, AAT also shows true substrate-like behaviour and cleavage without complex formation. Novel studies show that AAT, without forming complexes, inhibits the activity of gelatinase B (MMP9) and caspases-1 and -3 that play an essential role in cell apoptosis. AAT also inactivates the catalytic domain of matriptase, a cell surface serine protease involved in the activation of epithelial sodium channels. In addition, recent evidence has emerged on the ability of AAT to inhibit the matrix metalloprotease, ADAM-17 (Bergin et al., 2010) and aspartic-cysteine protease, calpain I (Al-Omari et al., 2011). Calpain I activity has been implicated in neutrophil apoptosis (Chen et al., 2006), chemotaxis (Lokuta et al., 2003) and adhesion (Wiemer et al., 2010). In fact, AAT inhibits neutrophil adhesion, chemotaxis (Al-Omari et al., 2011; Bergin et al., 2010) and apoptosis (Zhang et al., 2007). The mechanism behind these latter effects of AAT might be directly linked to its ability to inhibit calpain I activity.

So far, it is assumed that anti-inflammatory and immunomodulatory functions of AAT are dependent on its metastable native conformation (with inhibitory activity); however, this has not been proven. Earlier studies by Churg and collaborators have demonstrated that oxidized AAT (without elastase inhibitory activity) is effective in preventing neutrophil influx and lung tissue damage in a silica-induced inflammation model in mice (Churg et al., 2001). We also

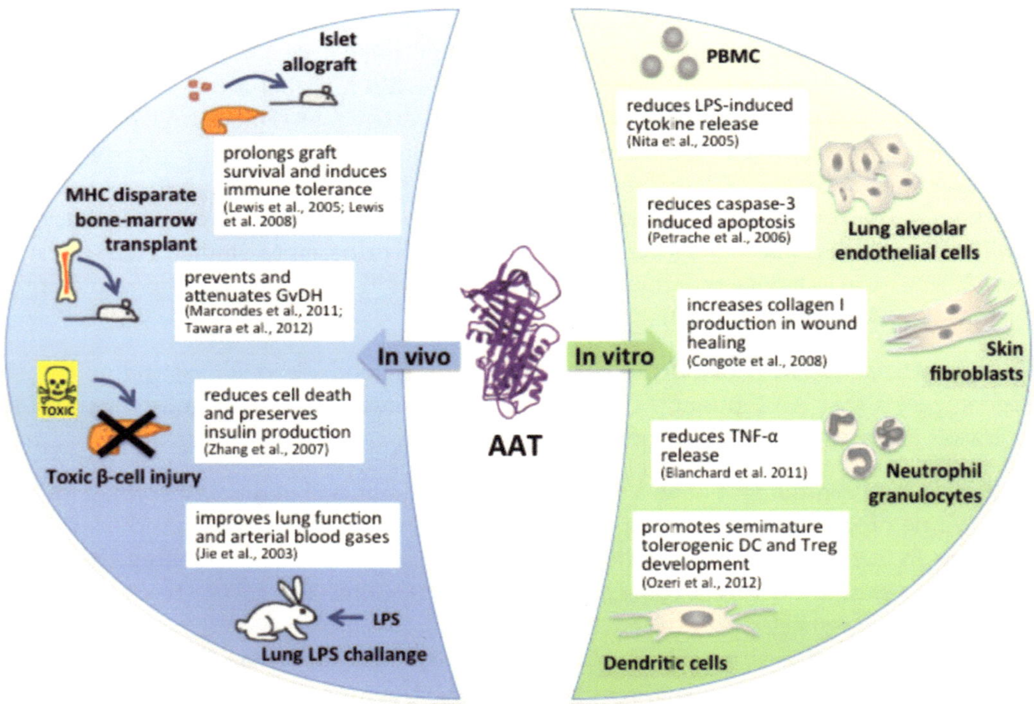

Figure 1. Selected anti-inflammatory and immunoregulatory activities of AAT.

reported that oxidized AAT (again without elastase inhibitory activity) reduces endotoxin-induced TNF-α, IL-8, MCP-1, and IL-1 release in human monocytes *in vitro* (Janciauskiene et al., 2004). We also found that the pattern of gene expression regulated in human primary lung endothelial cells by native and oxidized AAT was similar with neither inducing pro-inflammatory gene expression (Subramaniyam et al., 2008).

Moreover, a specific short carboxyl terminal peptide of AAT which doesn´t inhibit elastase is a more potent inhibitor of LPS-induced TNF-α and IL-8 production than native AAT (Amelinckx et al., 2011; Subramaniyam et al., 2006)

Recently, we examined the effects of plasma purified AAT in LPS-induced acute lung injury in wild-type (WT) and neutrophil elastase-deficient mice as well as in neutrophils isolated from the bone marrow of WT and elastase-deficient mice. Analyses of lung lavage fluids and tissues revealed that, regardless from the mouse strain, AAT induced a 50% decrease in LPS-induced neutrophil counts as well as a reduction in the lavage fluid levels of IL-8 and TNF-α. Furthermore, AAT inhibited the ability of LPS to increase TNF-α, DNA damage-inducible transcript 3 and X-box binding protein 1 gene expression in the lung parenchyma (Jonigk et al., PNAS, in press).

These findings provide clear evidence that inhibition of elastase is not the sole mechanism behind the anti-inflammatory and immunoregulatory activities of AAT. The responsible molecular mechanisms remain to be elucidated.

4. Interaction with other macromolecules and cell surface 'receptors' and signalling mechanisms

AAT shows the property to interact with other proteins. For example, in sera from patients with myeloma and Bence-Jones proteinemia complexes between AAT and the kappa light chain of immunoglobulins were detected (Laurell & Thulin, 1975). In plasma from diabetic subjects, complexes between AAT and factor Xia, AAT and heat shock protein-70 as well as AAT and glucose were detected (Murakami et al., 1993; Finotti & Pagetta, 2004; Hall et al., 1986). Moreover, complexes between AAT and immunoglobulin A have been detected in the sera and synovial fluid of patients with rheumatoid arthritis, systemic lupus erythematosus and ankylosing spondylitis (Adam & Bieth, 1996). Localization of AAT-low-density-lipoprotein (LDL) complexes in atherosclerotic lesions and enhanced degradation of AAT-LDL by macrophages suggested the involvement of the complex in atherogenesis (Mashiba et al., 2001).

Earlier studies have shown that cellular internalization and degradation of AAT-elastase-, or AAT-trypsin-complexes, but not of the native form of AAT, is mediated by serpin-enzyme complex (SEC) receptor (Perlmutter et al., 1990), low-density lipoprotein receptor related protein (Poller et al., 1995) and very-low-density lipoprotein receptor which require intact raft lipid environment (Wu & Gonias, 2005; Yoon et al., 2007).

Recent studies provide new evidence that clathrin-mediated endocytosis (Sohrab et al., 2009) and the caveolar pathway (Aldonyte et al., 2008) and Fc receptor(s) (Bergin et al., 2010) might be responsible for the interaction and entry of native AAT into the cell. Experimental studies have shown that various APPs, like C-reactive protein (CRP), interact with lipid rafts (Ji et al., 2009) and therefore, gave support for the hypothesis that APPs-lipid raft interaction may be a putative mechanism responsible for the diverse activities of APPs during inflammation.

Lipid rafts are dynamic assemblies of proteins and lipids that play a central role in various cellular processes, including membrane sorting and trafficking, cell polarization, and signal transduction (Baird et al., 1999; Janes et al., 2000; Zhu et al., 2006). Biochemical and cell-biological studies have identified cholesterol as a key factor determining raft and related structure (e.g., caveolae) stability and organization in mammalian cell membranes, and have shown that the equilibrium between free and raft cholesterol plays a critical role in lipid raft function and cell signalling (Golub et al., 2004; Gombos et al., 2006). Many proteins involved in signal transduction, such as Src family kinases, G proteins, growth factor receptors, mitogen-activated protein kinase and protein kinase C are predominantly found in lipid rafts, which act as signaling platforms by bringing together (i.e., colocalizing) various signaling components (Simons & Toomre, 2000).

Our studies on the putative role of lipid rafts and lipid raft cholesterol for AAT entry into monocytes revealed that exogenously added AAT becomes translocated into lipid rafts in the same fraction as the lipid raft marker flotillin (Slaughter et al., 2003; Subramaniyam et al., 2010). It is well documented that plasma membranes of mammalian cells contain a 30–50% molar fraction of cholesterol (Warnock et al., 1993), which is the dynamic glue for the lipid raft assembly (Simons & Toomre, 2000). Taken with the finding that exogenous AAT localizes in the lipid raft prompted us to examine whether altering the integrity of the lipid raft cholesterol would affect AAT-monocyte association. In fact, AAT association with monocytes was remarkably inhibited by various cholesterol depleting/efflux-stimulating agents such as nystatin, filipin, methyl-betacyclodextrin, oxidized low-density lipoprotein and high density lipoproteins, and conversely, enhanced by free cholesterol. We had previously identified that AAT can directly interact with free cholesterol in vitro (Janciauskiene & Eriksson, 1993). In support, we confirmed that AAT /monocyte association *per se* depletes lipid raft cholesterol as characterized by the activation of extracellular signal-regulated kinase 2, increased HMG-CoA reductase expression, formation of cytosolic lipid droplets, and a complete inhibition of oxidized low-density lipoprotein and oxidized phopspholipid uptake by monocytes (Subramaniyam et al., 2010).

Lipid rafts act as platforms, bringing together molecules essential for the activation of immune cells, but also separating such molecules when the conditions for activation are not appropriate (Ehrenstein et al., 2005). We hypothesize that AAT/ lipid raft interaction and cholesterol depletion contributes to re-organize membrane domains and facilitate the formation of compartment-specific signalling platforms. As a consequence, several events can occur intracellularly like transient release of calcium and Na^+/K^+-ATPase-EGFR-Src-caveolin-1 complex formation leading to an increased tyrosine phosphorylation of caveolin-1 and the activation of the Rac1-Cdc42-ERK cascade, and transient activation of hemoxygenase-1. It has been previously reported that exogenous AAT is rapidly internalized into the cells and is localized in the plasma membranes and in the cytoplasm (Sohrab et al., 2009). Whether internalized AAT is further trafficking to the interstitium or remains within the cells is

http://dx.doi.org/10.5772/56393

unknown. As a matter of fact, AAT is shown to interact with the transferrin receptor (Graziadei et al., 1994) which is constantly internalized via endocytic vesicles that fuse with early endosomes and returns to the plasma membrane through recycling endosomes (Harding et al., 1983). Thus it cannot be excluded that excess of internalized AAT trafficking occurs via transferrin receptor pathway.

Nevertheless, incorporation of AAT into membranes and transient depletion of cholesterol can affect recruitment of TLRs into lipid rafts subsequently desensitizing signalling by bacterial endotoxins and resulting in consequent reduction of the pro-inflammatory response. In support, human innate immune cells stimulated with bacterial lipopolysaccharide (LPS) in the presence of AAT show suppressed TNFα, IL-8, IL-12 and IL-1β, but enhanced IL-10 production (Figure 2) (Janciauskiene et al., 2004; Nita et al., 2005).

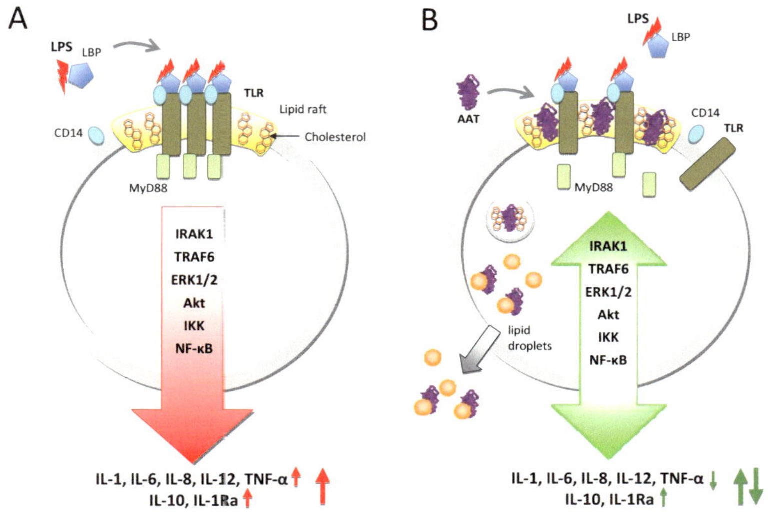

Figure 2. Hypothesis of the immune modulator effect of AAT. A: LPS signalling and cell activation; B: effects of AAT on LPS signalling and cell activation.

In general, this hypothesis provides the basis for future studies linking bioactivities of acute phase proteins to signalling pathways associated with lipid rafts. Lipid rafts are therapeutic targets for various diseases and studies on physiological significance of interaction between acute phase proteins and lipid rafts of great importance.

5. Diseases associated with AAT deficiency

The clinical relevance of AAT is highlighted in individuals with inherited deficiency in circulating AAT who have an increased susceptibility to early onset pulmonary emphysema, and liver as well as pancreatic diseases. The most interesting AAT variants associated with deficiency are the S and Z genes commonly found in Europeans. Both S and Z AAT result from single amino acid substitutions. In the S variant there is a substitution of a valine residue for glutamate at position 264 (Val264Glu) (Curiel et al., 1989). The Z mutation (Glu342Lys) results from the substitution of a positively charged lysine for a negatively charged glutamine at the base of the reactive centre. Severe ZZ deficiency of AAT is characterized by a decrease in serum AAT levels below a protective threshold of 11 mmol/L (Fregonese et al., 2008; Hubbard & Crystal, 1988) and is associated with increased but variable risk for the development of lung emphysema (Janciauskiene et al., 2010).

From retrospective studies we also know that up to 25% of those with severe AAT deficiency will suffer from liver cirrhosis and for liver cancer in late adulthood (Propst et al., 1994). Also heterozygous AAT deficiency is a cofactor in the development of chronic liver diseases (Kok et al., 2007). Adults with AAT deficiency–associated genotypes develop liver disease less frequently than pulmonary manifestations. However, AAT is a relevant cause for liver cirrhosis, after viral hepatitis, alcohol abuse, and chronic cholangitis. Other factors that can also predispose AAT-deficient individuals to liver disease are male sex and obesity (Bowlus et al., 2005).The underlying cause may be the intrahepatic accumulation of polymerized AAT molecules. The polymers of Z-mutant AAT can be identified in endoplasmic reticulum by the electron microscopy as diastase resistant inclusion bodies reacting positively with PAS-staining (Periodic acid-Schiff). Intracellular inclusion bodies in the liver have also been observed with other polymer-forming phenotypes of AAT deficiency (M_{malton} (52Phe del), and S_{iiyama} (Ser53Phe) (Tuder et al., 2010).

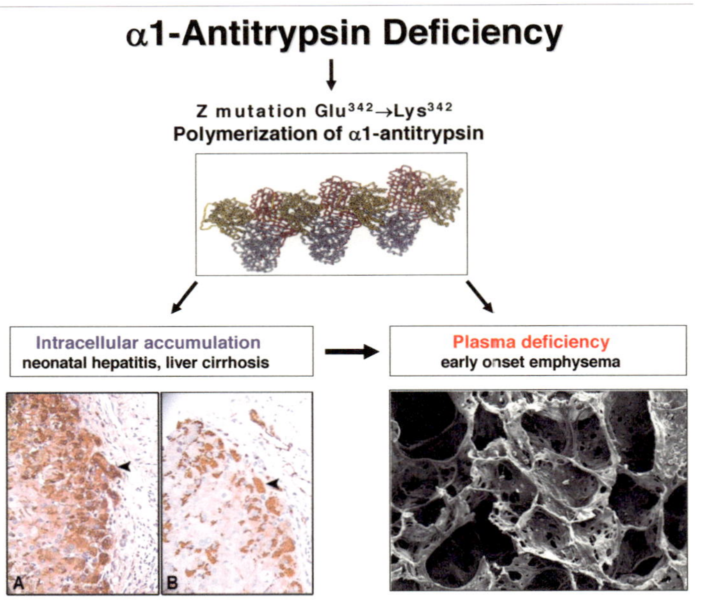

Figure 3. Schematic diagram depicting the role of polymers of α1-Antitrypsin (AAT) in the development of liver and lung diseases. A) AAT polymers stained with rabbit polyclonal antibody against human AAT, B) AAT polymers stained with mouse monoclonal ATZ11 antibody against human Z polymers.

Inherited AAT deficiency is occasionally associated with antiproteinase-3-associated vasculitis (Wegener's granulomatosis), necrotizing panniculitis and aneurysms of the abdominal aorta and brain arteries. AATD has also been associated with a number of other inflammatory diseases, although the association is only moderate or weak. These include bronchial asthma, bronchiectasis, rheumatoid arthritis, psoriasis, chronic urticaria, glomerulonephritis, pancreatitis and pancreatic tumors, multiple sclerosis, fibromyalgia and other conditions reported occasionally (Janciauskiene et al., 2011)

Remarkably, associations have been found between reduced plasma AAT levels and HIV-1 infection, hepatitis, diabetes mellitus, systemic vasculitis and necrotizing panniculitis (Lewis, 2012; Tuder et al., 2010).

5.1. AAT augmentation therapy

Given the concept of the protease/antiprotease imbalance role in causing emphysema, augmentation of circulating AAT was introduced 30 years ago to treat emphysema patients with severe ZZ deficiency of AAT. Augmentation therapy with human AAT has been performed for over a decade in the United States and in a number of European countries. Worldwide, more than 4,000 patients are currently receiving regular AAT substitution. Most patients receive weekly intravenous application of 3–5 g AAT (60 mg/kg body weight), which is derived from pooled human plasma. Patients with emphysema may be considered for augmentation if their serum concentration is below 0.8 g/L (≤ 11 μmol/L), if their post-bronchodilator FEV_1 is between 35% and 60% of predicted, or if their annual decline of FEV_1 is more than 100 mL (for review see (Mohanka et al., 2012))

Substitution therapy has been studied in a few clinical trials, and the evidence for its efficacy is limited. A last double-blind, placebo-controlled trial EXACTLE (the EXAcerbations and computed tomography (CT) scan as Lung Endpoints), was designed to explore the use of CT densitometry as an outcome measure for the assessment of the effect of AAT augmentation therapy on the progression of emphysema in individuals with inherited AAT deficiency (Stockley et al., 2010). This study showed that the rate of lung density decline was reduced by the intravenous augmentation therapy, and although the exacerbation frequency was unaltered by this treatment, a reduction in severity of exacerbations was observed.

To date fewer than 50 cases of panniculitis associated with various phenotypes of AAT deficiency have been reported (Filiang & Stoller, 2008). The clinical features that distinguish the AAT deficiency-associated panniculitis include higher frequency of ulceration, a vigorous neutrophilic response and histological evidence of both necrosis and elastin breakdown (Smith et al., 1989). In support of AAT deficiency as a contributor to the inflammatory pathogenesis of panniculitis, a few case reports provide evidence that the infusion of purified pooled human AAT induces a rapid clinical resolution of panniculitis (Gross et al., 2009; O'Riordan et al., 1997; Furey et al., 1996).

The putative association between AAT deficiency and vasculitis (Wegener's granulomatosis) is based on the fact that AAT deficiency variants occur more frequently among individuals with multisystem vascultitis (anti-neutrophilic cytoplasmic antibodies (C-ANCA) or antiprotease-3 (PR-3) and glomerulonephritis (Esnault et al., 1993; O'Donoghue et al., 1993; Montanelli et al., 2002). Moreover, since AAT plays an important role in inhibiting PR3, it has been suggested that AAT deficiency could trigger an autoimmune response due to increased extracellular exposure to PR3 (Esnault et al., 1997). Alternatively, although unproven, it is conceivable that circulating Z AAT polymers could prompt a vascular response.

5.2. New perspectives for use of the AAT augmentation therapy

Administration of exogenous human plasma-derived AAT is used in various animal models to test the value of AAT augmentation. Several studies report that administration of AAT results in a change from the pro-inflammatory to the anti-inflammatory pathways that is necessary for the resolution of inflammation. Cystic Fibrosis (CF) is a condition caused by a known gene defect which predisposes individuals to chronic lung inflammation and infection. To date work has demonstrated that CF neutrophils secrete abnormally high levels of the pro-inflammatory cytokines, such as IL-8 and TNFα, and proteolytic enzymes specifically elastase which not only causes lung parenchymal damage, but can also perpetuate a vicious cycle of inflammation by inducing expression of the neutrophil chemoattractant, IL-8, from bronchial epithelial cells. Therefore, the interest in the application of treatment with inhaled AAT in CF lung disease is discussed (Siekmeier, 2010)

Based on preclinical and clinical studies, it is suggested that AAT therapy can be successfully used for non-deficient individuals with Type-1 and Type-2 diabetes, acute myocardial infarction, rheumatoid arthritis, inflammatory bowel disease, cystic fibrosis, transplant rejection, graft-versus-host-disease and multiple sclerosis. AAT also appears to be antibacterial and an inhibitor of viral infections, such as influenza and HIV, and is currently evaluated in clinical trials for Type-1 diabetes, cystic fibrosis and graft-versus-host-disease (Blanco et al., 2011; Lewis, 2012). New experimental approaches show that AAT therapy might be an option for arthritis treatment in a combination with doxycycline (Grimstein et al., 2010)

Thus, AAT can be used as potential treatment for a broad spectrum of inflammatory and immune-mediated diseases. Future treatment developments include gene therapy (via injections of viral or non-viral vector systems carrying the SERPINA1-cDNA), strategies to inhibit intra-hepatic AAT polymerization by small chemicals and chaperons, and inhibition of neutrophil elastase by using small molecules. Inhaled application of AAT is currently under development by several companies.

6. Immunoregulatory properties of other APPs

The change in the concentrations of APPs is universally used to monitor the course of the disease, independently of its nature (Parra et al., 2006). However, specific APPs can also modify inflammatory responses. The spectrum of action of various APPs extends to regulation of leukocyte migration, adhesion and production of inflammatory mediators, control of ion channels and mucus secretion, and modulation of other host defence mechanisms (table 1).

http://dx.doi.org/10.5772/56393

Acute-phase protein	Main biological function
Proteins whose plasma concentration increase	
C-reactive protein (CRP)	Binding of phosphocholine (opsonin); immunoregulation
Alpha1-Acid Glycoprotein (AGP)	Carry lipophilic compounds; immunoregulation
Serum amyloid A (SAA)	Recruitment of immune cells; activation enzymes that degrade extracellular matrix
Fibronectin	Wound healing
Ferritin	Iron binding
Angiotensinogen	Renin substrate
Complement factors: C3, C4, C9, factor B, C1 inhibitor, C4b-binding protein, mannose-binding lectin	Enhancing phagocytosis of antigens, attracting macrophages and neutrophils, lysis membranes of foreign cells, clumping of antigen-bearing agents, altering the molecular structure of viruses
Coagulation and fibrinolysis factors: fibrinogen, plasminogen, tissue plasminogen activator, urokinase, protein S, vitronectin, plasminogen-activator inhibitor 1	Coagulation, degradation of blood clots, trapping invading microbes, chemotaxis
Ceruloplasmin	Contains copper, has histaminase-and ferroxidase-activity; scavenges Fe^{2+} and free radicals
Haptoglobin (Hp)	Binds haemoglobin; binds to CD_{11b}/CD_{18} integrines
Alpha1-acid glycoprotein (AGP)	Influences T-cell function; binds steroids
Interleukin1-receptor antagonist	modulates a variety of interleukin 1 related immune and inflammatory responses
Alpha1-Antitrypsin (AAT)	Inhibits proteolytic enzymes, immune-modulatory activity
Alpha1-Antichymotrypsin (ACT)	Inhibits proteolytic enzymes
Alpha2-macroglobulin	Inhibits proteolytic enzymes
Proteins whose concentration decrease	
Albumin	Regulates the osmotic pressure of blood
Transferrin	Carrier protein, immunoregulation
Transthyretin	Binds to aromatic compounds, carrier of retinol
Alpha-fetoprotein	Binds various cations, fatty acids and bilirubin
Alpha2-HS glycoprotein	Carrier protein, forms soluble complexes with calcium and phosphate
Thyroxine-binding globulin	Binds thyroid hormone

Table 1. Diverse functional activities of APPs.

7. Haptoglobin

Haptoglobin (Hp) is constitutively present in the plasma (normal plasma levels 0.3 to 3.0 mg/ml) and functions mainly as a scavenger protein for hemoglobin (Hb) that is released from erythrocytes. Hp-Hb complexes are rapidly cleared from the circulation predominantly in the liver (Kupfer cells) expressing the Hp-Hb receptor CD163 (Graversen et al., 2002). Hp not only prevents loss of Hb/iron by renal excretion and protects from iron-driven oxidative tissue damage, but also acts as a bacteriostatic protein. Hence, Hp restricts access of bacteria to iron that is essential for bacterial growth.

Plasma levels of Hp rise rapidly up to 2 to 5 folds during inflammation, specifically under conditions when there is an extensive amount of necrotic tissue in the wound. Like for other APPs, Hp synthesis is induced by various cytokines but also by ciliary neurotrophic factor. While IL-6 is the most efficient Hp inducer, IFN-γ blocks IL-6-induced Hp synthesis and TNF-β attenuates glucocorticoid-dependent expression of Hp (Baumann et al., 1990; Marinkovic & Baumann, 1990; Raynes et al., 1991; Yoshioka et al., 2002; Yu et al., 1999).

Although the liver is the major site of Hp expression, inducible expression of Hp is also found in lung, skin, spleen and kidney. This suggests that tissue levels of Hp are most likely regulated differently and vary from those in the blood (Abdullah et al., 2009). Therefore, locally expressed Hp, for example in the lungs, might be an important component of a local protection system with antioxidant, bacteriostatic and anti-inflammatory effects (Abdullah et al., 2012).

Hp influences almost every immune cell type of the innate as well as the adaptive immune response. As an example, binding of Hp-Hb to CD163 receptor on the monocytes and tissue macrophages (Kristiansen et al., 2001), induces anti-inflammatory and protective genes such as heme oxygenase-1 (HO-1) (Schaer et al., 2006). HO-1 is involved in heme catabolism that ends up with carbon monoxide, bilirubin and ferritin - all are known to exert potent anti-inflammatory and cytoprotective effects (Otterbein et al., 2003).

It has also been demonstrated that Hp inhibits respiratory burst in fMLP, arachindonic acid or opsonised zymosan-stimulated neutrophils (Oh et al., 1990). Moreover, Hp exerts inhibitory effects on fMLP-driven chemotaxis, and shows intracellular bactericidal activity against *E. coli.* (Rossbacher et al., 1999). Evidence exists for an intracellular uptake of Hp by peripheral blood neutrophils and monocytes via endocytosis and for the subsequent exocytosis of Hp following exposure to *Candida albicans* or TNF- α (Berkova et al., 1999; Wagner et al., 1996). Hp reduces LPS-induced pro-inflammatory effects by the selective suppression of TNF-α, IL-10 and IL-12 production *in vivo* and *in vivo*. The importance of anti-inflammatory and immune modulatory effects of Hp is confirmed by enhanced sensitivity of Hp knockout mice to LPS shock compared to wild type mice (Arredouani et al., 2005).

In addition to its effects on innate immunity, Hp also dampens adaptive immune response. It is a powerful inhibitor of the proliferative response of lymphocytes to phytohemagglutinin and concanavalin A, and depending on the concentration used Hp significantly inhibits or enhances mitogenesis in B-cells in response to LPS (Baseler & Burrell, 1983). Using highly purified human T lymphocytes Arredouani et al. presented evidence for a specific binding of Hp to resting and anti-CD3 stimulated CD4+ and CD8+ T cells and for a direct anti-proliferative effect of Hp on T lymphocytes (Arredouani et al., 2003).

Further evidence for the high importance of Hp as anti-oxidative and immunoregulatory compound arises from the existence of different Hp subtypes and their influence on different pathologies. Hp gene has been studied as a candidate gene for rheumatoid arthritis, systemic lupus erythematosus, primary sclerosing cholangitis, inflammatory bowel disease and diabetes mellitus type 2 (Marquez et al., 2012).

In human two allels code for Hp1 and Hp2 proteins resulting in Hp1-1, Hp2-2 homozygous and Hp2-1 heterozygous genotypes. Clinical studies show that Hp2-2 individuals suffering from diabetes mellitus have a higher risk of vascular complications, especially diabetic nephropathy, compared to Hp2-1 and Hp1-1 individuals (Asleh & Levy, 2005). Epidemiological data also show that Hp2-2 genotype is a major determinant of susceptibility to diabetic cardiovascular disease (Levy et al., 2010).

Functional differences between Hp1-1 and Hp2-2 on molecular level can be in part explained by the finding that the Hp1-1-Hb complex is endocytosed more rapidly by the CD163 pathway than Hp2-2-Hb. This results in a more effective clearance of Hb and less oxidative stress in Hp1-1 individuals (Asleh et al., 2003). Moreover, Hp2-2 individuals show greater immunological reactivity including higher antibody titers after vaccination compared to Hp1-1 and Hp2-1 individuals (Nevo & Sutton, 1968). When compare to Hp2-2-Hb, Hp1-1-Hb is related to a much greater production of anti-inflammatory cytokines, therefore, Hp1-1Hp results in a more Th2 directed balance between Th1 (inflammatory) and Th2 (anti-inflammatory) T helper cells. Recent findings provide evidence that Hp1-1 individuals are better protected against oxidative stress and Hp1-1 seems to have higher immunomodulatory effects than Hp 2-2 (Guetta et al., 2007).

8. Alpha-1-acid glycoprotein

Alpha-1-acid glycoprotein (AGP) also known as orosomucoid (ORM) is a heavily glycosylated (45 %) protein (Schmid et al., 1977) APG belongs to the immunocalin family, a lipocalin subfamily. Whereas the lipocalins function as carriers for small hydrophobic compounds, the immunocalins were shown to modulate inflammatory and immune responses (Logdberg & Wester, 2000; Hochepied et al., 2003). Though, the main biologic function of AGP remains unclear. Indeed, APG was found to be a major carrier for neutral and basic drugs in the blood (Kremer et al., 1988). Evidence also exists supporting a role for AGP in the maintenance of normal capillary permeability and selectivity by binding to the capillary vessel wall putatively as part of the glycocalyx, a dynamic endothelial surface layer of glycosaminoglycans, proteoglycans and absorbed plasma proteins (Curry et al., 1989; Fournier et al., 2000; Pries et al., 2000). Moreover, AGP stabilizes the biological activity of plasminogen activator inhibitor-1 (Smolarczyk et al., 2005).

AGP is a positive acute phase protein that under normal conditions circulates in human plasma at a concentration of 0.6 -1.2 mg/ml and rises up to 2- to 7-fold during acute phase response (Colombo et al., 2006; Kremer et al., 1988). Besides the liver, a main source for the circulating AGP levels, production of AGP occurs in human microvascular endothelial cells, pneumocytes, alveolar macrophages, neutrophils, monocytes and B and T lymphocytes (Sirica et al., 1979; Sorensson et al., 1999; Crestani et al., 1998; Martinez Cordero et al., 2008; Fournier et al.,

1999; Theilgaard-Monch et al., 2005; Rahman et al., 2008; Gahmberg & Andersson, 1978; Dirienzo et al., 1987). Hepatic AGP expression is induced by the IL-1β, IL-6 and TNF-α and inhibited by the growth hormone (Barraud et al., 1996; Mejdoubi et al., 1999).

The immunomodulatory activities of AGP are specifically directed against exaggerated inflammatory response to tissue damage. For example, AGP in a concentration-dependent manner regulates neutrophil chemotactic migration and superoxide generation (Costello et al., 1984; Hochepied et al., 2003; Laine et al., 1990). AGP also inhibits monocyte chemotaxis and diminishes cellular leakage caused by histamine and bradykinin. Moreover, AGP induces secretion of soluble TNFα receptor and IL-1 receptor antagonist from peripheral blood monocytes. (Tilg et al., 1993; Samak et al., 1982; Muchitsch et al., 1996).

The effects of AGP on lymphocytes are mainly immunosuppressive. AGP significantly suppresses induced synthesis of IL-2 and proliferation of lymphocytes (Chiu et al., 1977; Elg et al., 1997). Notably, different glycan variants of AGP show different degrees of inhibition of lymphocyte proliferation (Bennett & Schmid, 1980). The Con A non-reactive fraction of AGP (AGP-A) inhibits anti-CD3 stimulated lymphocyte proliferation stronger than Con A reactive AGP forms emphasizing the importance of the carbohydrate moiety of AGP (Pos et al., 1990).

In vivo AGP has been found to protect mice against TNF-α induced lethal shock but not from LPS-induced lethality or Fas-mediated cell death in lethal hepatitis. These findings imply that the protecting effects of AGP are, most likely, TNF-α -specific (Muchitsch et al., 1998; Van Molle et al., 1999).

Pro-inflammatory and immuno-stimulatory effects of AGP have been described, too. Previous studies demonstrated that AGP activates monocytes to produce IL-1β, IL-6, IL-12, TNF-α and tissue factor (Su & Yeh, 1996; Tilg et al., 1993). Moreover, AGP has found to potentiate the effect of suboptimal concentrations of LPS to induce IL-1β, IL-6 and TNF-α in peritoneal and alveolar macrophages (Boutten et al., 1992). Nakamura and collaborators presented evidence that monocytes stimulated with inflammatory cytokines produce AGP and suggested that high expression of AGP may potentially create a positive feedback loop for further production of IL-1β (Nakamura et al., 1993). The observation that AGP-induced secretion of TNFα can be inhibited by protein tyrosine kinase inhibitors led to the proposal that AGP involves tyrosine kinase signalling pathway (Su et al., 1999). This is in line with the finding that AGP binds to chemokine receptor CCR5 on macrophages and signals via tyrosine kinases (Atemezem et al., 2001). In neutrophil models AGP interacts with lectin-like receptors (Siglecs), Siglec-5 and/or Siglec-14, directly induces an intracellular calcium rise and regulates expression of L-selectin (Gunnarsson et al., 2007).

Recently, it has been reported that AGP up-regulates the expression of the Hb scavenger receptor CD163 on monocytic cells *in vitro* (Komori et al., 2012). *In vivo*, in the phenylhydrazine-induced hemolysis mice model AGP induced CD163 expression with a subsequent increase in Hb clearance and reduced oxidative stress. The effect of AGP on CD163 expression seems to be indirect and mediated by the IL-6 and IL-10, known inducers of CD163. According to Komori and co-workers AGP induces CD163 expression via the TLR4/CD14 pathway (Komori et al., 2012).

http://dx.doi.org/10.5772/56393

Taken together AGP seems to exhibit both pro- and anti-inflammatory effects. The resulting net function of AGP most likely depends on contextual factors, e.g. interacting cell type, additional stimuli, inflammatory status of the host.

9. C-reactive protein

Human C-reactive protein (CRP) belongs to a family of pentraxins (Myles et al., 1990) and is composed of five identical 23 kDa subunits (protomers), linked together non-covalently to form pentameric CRP. The liver is the main source for circulating CRP. Hepatic secretion of CRP is primarily regulated by IL-6 and IL-1 (Weinhold et al., 1997; Zhang et al., 1995). Plasma CRP is a highly dynamic protein with a concentration range from 0.05 to 500 μg/ml (Shine et al., 1981; Pepys & Hirschfield, 2003). Plasma CRP levels rise up to 10.000-fold in response to acute tissue injury or inflammation and decline rapidly due to a relatively short half-life (about 19 hours) (Macintyre et al., 1982; Claus et al., 1976; Vigushin et al., 1993). Cardiovascular disease is correlated to chronic inflammation and serum CRP above 3 μg/ml is a good predictive of increased risk for the disease (Black et al., 2004).

Both *in vitro* and *in vivo* CRP exists in a monomeric form (mCRP) with a molecular weight of 23 kDa, too (Taylor & van den Berg, 2007). The pentameric native form of CRP (nCRP) is usually found in the plasma whereas the momomeric form of CRP (mCRP) is present in tissues and at sites of inflammation (Diehl et al., 2000; Potempa et al., 1987; Rees et al., 1988). pCRP also undergoes conformational rearrangement in the absence of calcium and dissociates into mCRP (Eisenhardt et al., 2009). The modified CRP isoform is generated *in vivo* when pCRP binds to damaged membrane surfaces such as activated platelets, apoptotic microparticles (Habersberger et al., 2012), liposomes containing lysophosphatidylcholine (Volanakis & Narkates, 1981), and oxidized but not native low-density lipoprotein (Chang et al., 2002). Modified CRP displays an antigenicity that is distinct from pCRP. In fact, modified CRP may exist as aggregates of mCRP on cell membrane surfaces (Ji et al., 2007).

One critical function of modified CRP is binding to C1q and activation of the immune system's complement cascade (Ji et al., 2006). In addition to its roles in the regulation of classical and alternative complement pathways, CRP has been shown to interact with ficolin-2 (Ng et al., 2007). Recent study has shown that infection-induced local inflammatory conditions trigger a strong interaction between CRP and ficolin-2; this elicits complement amplification and enhances antimicrobial activation of the classical and lectin pathways (Zhang et al., 2009).

Despite evidence that modified CRP is more strongly associated with inflammation (Zouki et al., 2001) current CRP diagnostics are unable to distinguish between the common isoforms.

Taken together, physiological function of CRP is not fully understood. The most reproducible observations indicate that CRP contributes to innate immunity against bacterial infections like pneumococci (Horowitz et al., 1987). Experimental data provide evidence that transgenic mice over-expressing human CRP are more resistant to *Pneumococci* sepsis than wild-type mice (Szalai et al., 1995). Indeed, CRP is expressed by respiratory epithelial cells and CRP concentrations in secretions from both inflamed and non-inflamed human respiratory tract are sufficiently high for an antimicrobial effect. This suggests that CRP is involved in the bacterial clearance in the respiratory tract (Gould & Weiser, 2001).

Recent findings lend experimental support to the hypothesis that biological activities of CRP might be dependent on both, its molecular form and the property to interact with plasma membrane lipid microdomains (Ji et al., 2009).

For example, CRP and two CRP derived peptides, CRP(174-185) and CRP(201-206), but not peptide CRP(77-82) are capable of diminishing attachment of human neutrophils to LPS-stimulated human endothelial cells and consequently limiting leukocyte traffic into inflamed tissues (Zouki et al., 1997). CRP as well as the two peptides rapidly downregulate the expression of L-selectin on the neutrophil surface.

In summary, CRP is used as an indicator of disease outcome and to monitor the disease course. CRP is measured objectively and affordably in clinical practice worldwide.

10. Conclusions

In this chapter we have shown that AAT, only one among many APPs, holds tremendous potential as an anti-inflammatory and immuno-modulatory protein.

Several *in vitro* and *in vivo* studies have been published in which a specific APP switched the pro-inflammatory to the anti-inflammatory pathways necessary for the resolution of inflammation. Although the physiological roles of APPs are not completely understood, existing findings provide evidence that APPs act on a variety of cells involved in early and late stages of inflammation and that their effects are time, concentration and molecular conformation-dependent. It cannot be excluded that these proteins may have more common characteristics and biological effects, however the lack of high quality purified endotoxin or other contaminant free proteins limits current understanding.

The mechanisms of action for the APPs are still being investigated, however, there remain a number of challenges to face in the development of APPs as a true anti-inflammatory therapeutic agents and diagnostic markers.

Author details

S. Janciauskiene, S. Wrenger and T. Welte

Department of Respiratory Medicine, Hannover Medical School, Hannover, Germany

References

[1] Abdullah, M, et al. (2012). Pulmonary haptoglobin and CD163 are functional immunoregulatory elements in the human lung. *Respiration* , 83, 61-73.

[2] Abdullah, M, et al. (2009). Expression of the acute phase protein haptoglobin in human lung cancer and tumor-free lung tissues. *Pathol Res Pract* , 205, 639-647.

[3] Adam, C, et al. (1996). Inhibition of neutrophil elastase by the alpha1-proteinase inhibitor-immunoglobulin A complex. *FEBS Lett* , 385, 201-204.

[4] Al-omari, M, et al. (2011). Acute-phase protein alpha1-antitrypsin inhibits neutrophil calpain I and induces random migration. *Mol Med* , 17, 865-874.

[5] Aldonyte, R, et al. (2008). Endothelial alpha-1-antitrypsin attenuates cigarette smoke induced apoptosis in vitro. *COPD* , 5, 153-162.

[6] Amelinckx, A, et al. (2011). Neutrophil Chemotaxis Induced by Molecular Modifications of Alpha-1 Antitrypsin (AAT) in COPD Subjects with and without AAT Deficiency. *Am J Respir Crit Care Med* 183, A2429.

[7] Arredouani, M, et al. (2003). Haptoglobin directly affects T cells and suppresses T helper cell type 2 cytokine release. *Immunology* , 108, 144-151.

[8] Arredouani, M. S, et al. (2005). Haptoglobin dampens endotoxin-induced inflammatory effects both in vitro and in vivo. *Immunology* , 114, 263-271.

[9] Asleh, R, et al. (2005). In vivo and in vitro studies establishing haptoglobin as a major susceptibility gene for diabetic vascular disease. *Vasc Health Risk Manag* , 1, 19-28.

[10] Asleh, R, et al. (2003). Genetically determined heterogeneity in hemoglobin scavenging and susceptibility to diabetic cardiovascular disease. *Circ Res* , 92, 1193-1200.

[11] Atemezem, A, et al. (2001). Human alpha1-acid glycoprotein binds to CCR5 expressed on the plasma membrane of human primary macrophages. *Biochem J* , 356, 121-128.

[12] Baird, B, et al. (1999). How does the plasma membrane participate in cellular signaling by receptors for immunoglobulin E? *Biophys Chem* , 82, 109-119.

[13] Barraud, B, et al. (1996). Effects of insulin, dexamethasone and cytokines on alpha 1-acid glycoprotein gene expression in primary cultures of normal rat hepatocytes. *Inflammation* , 20, 191-202.

[14] Baseler, M. W, et al. (1983). Purification of haptoglobin and its effects on lymphocyte and alveolar macrophage responses. *Inflammation* , 7, 387-400.

[15] Baumann, H, et al. (1990). Distinct regulation of the interleukin-1 and interleukin-6 response elements of the rat haptoglobin gene in rat and human hepatoma cells. *Mol Cell Biol* , 10, 5967-5976.

[16] Bennett, M, et al. (1980). Immunosuppression by human plasma alpha 1-acid glycoprotein: importance of the carbohydrate moiety. *Proc Natl Acad Sci U S A* , 77, 6109-6113.

[17] Bergin, D. A, et al. (2010). alpha-1 Antitrypsin regulates human neutrophil chemotaxis induced by soluble immune complexes and IL-8. *J Clin Invest* , 120, 4236-4250.

[18] Berkova, N, et al. (1999). TNF-induced haptoglobin release from human neutrophils: pivotal role of the TNF receptor. *J Immunol* 162, 6226-6232., 55.

[19] Berman, M. B, et al. (1973). Corneal ulceration and the serum antiproteases. I. Alpha 1-antitrypsin. *Invest Ophthalmol* , 12, 759-770.

[20] Black, S, et al. (2004). C-reactive Protein. *J Biol Chem* , 279, 48487-48490.

[21] Blanchard, V, et al. (2011). N-glycosylation and biological activity of recombinant human alpha1-antitrypsin expressed in a novel human neuronal cell line. *Biotechnol Bioeng* , 108, 2118-2128.

[22] Blanco, I, et al. (2011). Efficacy of alphaantitrypsin augmentation therapy in conditions other than pulmonary emphysema. *Orphanet J Rare Dis* 6, 14., 1.

[23] Borregaard, N, et al. (1992). Stimulus-dependent secretion of plasma proteins from human neutrophils. *J Clin Invest* , 90, 86-96.

[24] Bosco, D, et al. (2005). Expression and secretion of alpha1-proteinase inhibitor are regulated by proinflammatory cytokines in human pancreatic islet cells. *Diabetologia* , 48, 1523-1533.

[25] Boskovic, G, et al. (1997). Retinol and retinaldehyde specifically increase alphaproteinase inhibitor in the human cornea. *Biochem J* 322 (Pt 3), 751-756., 1.

[26] Boskovic, G, et al. (1998). Local control of alpha1-proteinase inhibitor levels: regulation of alpha1-proteinase inhibitor in the human cornea by growth factors and cytokines. *Biochim Biophys Acta* , 1403, 37-46.

[27] Boutten, A, et al. (1992). Alpha 1-acid glycoprotein potentiates lipopolysaccharide-induced secretion of interleukin-1 beta, interleukin-6 and tumor necrosis factor-alpha by human monocytes and alveolar and peritoneal macrophages. *Eur J Immunol* , 22, 2687-2695.

[28] Boutten, A, et al. (1998). Oncostatin M is a potent stimulator of alpha1-antitrypsin secretion in lung epithelial cells: modulation by transforming growth factor-beta and interferon-gamma. *Am J Respir Cell Mol Biol* , 18, 511-520.

[29] Bowlus, C. L, et al. (2005). Factors associated with advanced liver disease in adults with alpha1-antitrypsin deficiency. *Clin Gastroenterol Hepatol* , 3, 390-396.

[30] Chang, M. K, et al. (2002). C-reactive protein binds to both oxidized LDL and apoptotic cells through recognition of a common ligand: Phosphorylcholine of oxidized phospholipids. *Proc Natl Acad Sci U S A* , 99, 13043-13048.

[31] Chen, H. C, et al. (2006). Tumor necrosis factor-alpha induces caspase-independent cell death in human neutrophils via reactive oxidants and associated with calpain activity. *J Biomed Sci* , 13, 261-273.

[32] Chiu, K. M, et al. (1977). Interactions of alpha1-acid glycoprotein with the immune system. I. Purification and effects upon lymphocyte responsiveness. *Immunology* , 32, 997-1005.

[33] Chowanadisai, W, et al. (2002). Alpha(1)-antitrypsin and antichymotrypsin in human milk: origin, concentrations, and stability. *Am J Clin Nutr* , 76, 828-833.

[34] Churg, A, et al. (2001). Alpha-1-antitrypsin and a broad spectrum metalloprotease inhibitor, RS113456, have similar acute anti-inflammatory effects. *Lab Invest* , 81, 1119-1131.

[35] Claus, D. R, et al. (1976). Radioimmunoassay of human C-reactive protein and levels in normal sera. *J Lab Clin Med* , 87, 120-128.

[36] Clemmensen, S. N, et al. (2011). Alpha-1-antitrypsin is produced by human neutrophil granulocytes and their precursors and liberated during granule exocytosis. *Eur J Haematol* , 86, 517-530.

[37] Colombo, S, et al. (2006). Orosomucoid (alpha1-acid glycoprotein) plasma concentration and genetic variants: effects on human immunodeficiency virus protease inhibitor clearance and cellular accumulation. *Clin Pharmacol Ther* , 80, 307-318.

[38] Congote, L. F, et al. (2008). Comparison of the effects of serpin A1, a recombinant serpin A1-IGF chimera and serpin A1 C-terminal peptide on wound healing. *Peptides* , 29, 39-46.

[39] Costello, M. J, et al. (1984). Inhibition of neutrophil activation by alpha1-acid glycoprotein. *Clin Exp Immunol* , 55, 465-472.

[40] Crestani, B, et al. (1998). Inducible expression of the alpha1-acid glycoprotein by rat and human type II alveolar epithelial cells. *J Immunol* , 160, 4596-4605.

[41] Curiel, D. T, et al. (1989). Serum alpha 1-antitrypsin deficiency associated with the common S-type (Glu264----Val) mutation results from intracellular degradation of alpha 1-antitrypsin prior to secretion. *J Biol Chem* , 264, 10477-10486.

[42] Curry, F. E, et al. (1989). Modulation of microvessel wall charge by plasma glycoprotein orosomucoid. *Am J Physiol* 257, H, 1354-1359.

[43] Daemen, M. A, et al. (2000). Functional protection by acute phase proteins alpha(1)-acid glycoprotein and alpha(1)-antitrypsin against ischemia/reperfusion injury by preventing apoptosis and inflammation. *Circulation* , 102, 1420-1426.

[44] Diehl, E. E, et al. (2000). Immunohistochemical localization of modified C-reactive protein antigen in normal vascular tissue. *Am J Med Sci* , 319, 79-83.

[45] Dirienzo, W, et al. (1987). Alpha 1-acid glycoprotein (alpha 1-AGP) on the membrane of human lymphocytes: possible involvement in cellular activation. *Immunol Lett* , 15, 167-170.

[46] Ehrenstein, M. R, et al. (2005). Statins for atherosclerosis--as good as it gets? *N Engl J Med* , 352, 73-75.

[47] Eisenhardt, S. U, et al. (2009). Monomeric C-reactive protein generation on activated platelets: the missing link between inflammation and atherothrombotic risk. *Trends Cardiovasc Med* , 19, 232-237.

[48] Elg, S. A, et al. (1997). Alpha-1 acid glycoprotein is an immunosuppressive factor found in ascites from ovaria carcinoma. *Cancer* , 80, 1448-1456.

[49] Esnault, V. L, et al. (1997). Alpha-1-antitrypsin phenotyping in ANCA-associated diseases: one of several arguments for protease/antiprotease imbalance in systemic vasculitis. *Exp Clin Immunogenet* , 14, 206-213.

[50] Esnault, V. L, et al. (1993). Alpha 1-antitrypsin genetic polymorphism in ANCA-positive systemic vasculitis. *Kidney Int* , 43, 1329-1332.

[51] Faust, D, et al. (2001). Butyrate and the cytokine-induced alpha1-proteinase inhibitor release in intestinal epithelial cells. *Eur J Clin Invest* , 31, 1060-1063.

[52] Finotti, P, et al. (2004). A heat shock protein70 fusion protein with alpha1-antitrypsin in plasma of type 1 diabetic subjects. *Biochem Biophys Res Commun* , 315, 297-305.

[53] Fournier, T, et al. (1999). Inducible expression and regulation of the alpha 1-acid glycoprotein gene by alveolar macrophages: prostaglandin E2 and cyclic AMP act as new positive stimuli. *J Immunol* , 163, 2883-2890.

[54] Fournier, T, et al. (2000). Alpha-1-acid glycoprotein. *Biochim Biophys Acta* , 1482, 157-171.

[55] Fregonese, L, et al. (2008). Alpha-1 antitrypsin Null mutations and severity of emphysema. *Respir Med* , 102, 876-884.

[56] Furey, N. L, et al. (1996). Treatment of alpha-antitrypsin deficiency, massive edema, and panniculitis with alpha-1 protease inhibitor. *Ann Intern Med* 125, 699., 1.

[57] Gahmberg, C. G, et al. (1978). Leukocyte surface origin of human alpha1-acid glycoprotein (orosomucoid). *J Exp Med* , 148, 507-521.

[58] Geboes, K, et al. (1982). Morphological identification of alpha-I-antitrypsin in the human small intestine. *Histopathology* , 6, 55-60.

[59] Gettins, P. G. (2002). Serpin structure, mechanism, and function. *Chem Rev* , 102, 4751-4804.

[60] Golub, T, et al. (2004). Spatial and temporal control of signaling through lipid rafts. *Curr Opin Neurobiol* , 14, 542-550.

[61] Gombos, I, et al. (2006). Cholesterol and sphingolipids as lipid organizers of the immune cells' plasma membrane: their impact on the functions of MHC molecules, effector T-lymphocytes and T-cell death. *Immunol Lett* , 104, 59-69.

[62] Gould, J. M, et al. (2001). Expression of C-reactive protein in the human respiratory tract. *Infect Immun* , 69, 1747-1754.

[63] Graversen, J. H, et al. (2002). CD163: a signal receptor scavenging haptoglobin-hemoglobin complexes from plasma. *Int J Biochem Cell Biol* , 34, 309-314.

[64] Graziadei, I, et al. (1994). The acute-phase protein alpha 1-antitrypsin inhibits growth and proliferation of human early erythroid progenitor cells (burst-forming units-erythroid) and of human erythroleukemic cells (K562) in vitro by interfering with transferrin iron uptake. *Blood* , 83, 260-268.

[65] Graziadei, I, et al. (1997). Unidirectional upregulation of the synthesis of the major iron proteins, transferrin-receptor and ferritin, in HepG2 cells by the acute-phase protein alpha1-antitrypsin. *J Hepatol* , 27, 716-725.

[66] Grimstein, C, et al. (2010). Combination of alpha-1 antitrypsin and doxycycline suppresses collagen-induced arthritis. *J Gene Med* , 12, 35-44.

[67] Gross, B, et al. (2009). New Findings in PiZZ alpha1-antitrypsin deficiency-related panniculitis. Demonstration of skin polymers and high dosing requirements of intravenous augmentation therapy. *Dermatology* , 218, 370-375.

[68] Guetta, J, et al. (2007). Haptoglobin genotype modulates the balance of Th1/Th2 cytokines produced by macrophages exposed to free hemoglobin. *Atherosclerosis* , 191, 48-53.

[69] Gunnarsson, P, et al. (2007). The acute-phase protein alpha 1-acid glycoprotein (AGP) induces rises in cytosolic Ca2+ in neutrophil granulocytes via sialic acid binding immunoglobulin-like lectins (siglecs). *FASEB J* , 21, 4059-4069.

[70] Habersberger, J, et al. (2012). Circulating microparticles generate and transport monomeric C-reactive protein in patients with myocardial infarction. *Cardiovasc Res*

[71] Hall, P, et al. (1986). Functional activities and nonenzymatic glycosylation of plasma proteinase inhibitors in diabetes. *Clin Chim Acta* , 160, 55-62.

[72] Harding, C, et al. (1983). Receptor-mediated endocytosis of transferrin and recycling of the transferrin receptor in rat reticulocytes. *J Cell Biol* , 97, 329-339.

[73] Hochepied, T, et al. (2003). Alpha(1)-acid glycoprotein: an acute phase protein with inflammatory and immunomodulating properties. *Cytokine Growth Factor Rev* , 14, 25-34.

[74] Horowitz, J, et al. (1987). Blood clearance of Streptococcus pneumoniae by C-reactive protein. *J Immunol* , 138, 2598-2603.

[75] Huang, C. M. (2004). Comparative proteomic analysis of human whole saliva. *Arch Oral Biol* , 49, 951-962.

[76] Hubbard, R. C, et al. (1988). Alpha-1-antitrypsin augmentation therapy for alpha-1-antitrypsin deficiency. *Am J Med* , 84, 52-62.

[77] Janciauskiene, S. (2001). Conformational properties of serine proteinase inhibitors (serpins) confer multiple pathophysiological roles. *Biochim Biophys Acta* , 1535, 221-235.

[78] Janciauskiene, S, et al. (1993). In vitro complex formation between cholesterol and alpha 1-proteinase inhibitor. *FEBS Lett* , 316, 269-272.

[79] Janciauskiene, S, et al. (2004). Inhibition of lipopolysaccharide-mediated human monocyte activation, in vitro, by alpha1-antitrypsin. *Biochem Biophys Res Commun* , 321, 592-600.

[80] Janciauskiene, S, et al. (2010). Plasma levels of TIMP-1 are higher in year-old individuals with severe alpha1-antitrypsin deficiency. *Thorax* 65, 937., 34.

[81] Janciauskiene, S, et al. (1996). Immunochemical and functional properties of biliary alpha-1-antitrypsin. *Scand J Clin Lab Invest* , 56, 597-608.

[82] Janciauskiene, S. M, et al. (2011). The discovery of alpha1-antitrypsin and its role in health and disease. *Respir Med* , 105, 1129-1139.

[83] Janes, P. W, et al. (2000). The role of lipid rafts in T cell antigen receptor (TCR) signalling. *Semin Immunol* , 12, 23-34.

[84] Ji, S. R, et al. (2009). Monomeric C-reactive protein activates endothelial cells via interaction with lipid raft microdomains. *FASEB J* , 23, 1806-1816.

[85] Ji, S. R, et al. (2006). Effect of modified C-reactive protein on complement activation: a possible complement regulatory role of modified or monomeric C-reactive protein in atherosclerotic lesions. *Arterioscler Thromb Vasc Biol* , 26, 935-941.

[86] Ji, S. R, et al. (2007). Cell membranes and liposomes dissociate C-reactive protein (CRP) to form a new, biologically active structural intermediate: mCRP(m). *FASEB J* , 21, 284-294.

[87] Jie, Z, et al. (2003). Protective effects of alpha 1-antitrypsin on acute lung injury in rabbits induced by endotoxin. *Chin Med J (Engl)* , 116, 1678-1682.

[88] Johansson, B, et al. (2001). Alpha-1-antitrypsin is present in the specific granules of human eosinophilic granulocytes. *Clin Exp Allergy* , 31, 379-386.

[89] Kalsheker, N, et al. (2002). Gene regulation of the serine proteinase inhibitors alpha1-antitrypsin and alpha1-antichymotrypsin. *Biochem Soc Trans* , 30, 93-98.

[90] Knoell, D. L, et al. (1998). Alpha 1-antitrypsin and protease complexation is induced by lipopolysaccharide, interleukin-1beta, and tumor necrosis factor-alpha in monocytes. *Am J Respir Crit Care Med* , 157, 246-255.

[91] Kok, K. F, et al. (2007). Heterozygous alpha-I antitrypsin deficiency as a co-factor in the development of chronic liver disease: a review. *Neth J Med* , 65, 160-166.

[92] Komori, H, et al. (2012). alpha1-Acid Glycoprotein Up-regulates CD163 via TLR4/CD14 Protein Pathway: POSSIBLE PROTECTION AGAINST HEMOLYSIS-INDUCED OXIDATIVE STRESS. *J Biol Chem* , 287, 30688-30700.

[93] Kremer, J. M, et al. (1988). Drug binding to human alpha-1-acid glycoprotein in health and disease. *Pharmacol Rev* , 40, 1-47.

[94] Kristiansen, M, et al. (2001). Identification of the haemoglobin scavenger receptor. *Nature* , 409, 198-201.

[95] Laine, E, et al. (1990). Modulation of human polymorphonuclear neutrophil functions by alpha 1-acid glycoprotein. *Inflammation* , 14, 1-9.

[96] Laurell, C. B, et al. (1975). Thiol-disulfide interchange in the binding of bence jones proteins to alpha-antitrypsin, prealbumin, and albumin. *J Exp Med* , 141, 453-465.

[97] Levy, A. P, et al. (2010). Haptoglobin: basic and clinical aspects. *Antioxid Redox Signal* , 12, 293-304.

[98] Lewis, E. C. (2012). Expanding the Clinical Indications for Alpha-Antitrypsin Therapy. *Mol Med*, 1.

[99] Lewis, E. C, et al. (2008). alpha1-Antitrypsin monotherapy induces immune tolerance during islet allograft transplantation in mice. *Proc Natl Acad Sci U S A* , 105, 16236-16241.

[100] Lewis, E. C, et al. (2005). Alpha1-antitrypsin monotherapy prolongs islet allograft survival in mice. *Proc Natl Acad Sci U S A* , 102, 12153-12158.

[101] Logdberg, L, et al. (2000). Immunocalins: a lipocalin subfamily that modulates immune and inflammatory responses. *Biochim Biophys Acta* , 1482, 284-297.

[102] Lokuta, M. A, et al. (2003). Calpain regulates neutrophil chemotaxis. *Proc Natl Acad Sci U S A* , 100, 4006-4011.

[103] Macintyre, S. S, et al. (1982). Biosynthesis of C-reactive protein. *Ann N Y Acad Sci* , 389, 76-87.

[104] Marcondes, A. M, et al. (2011). Inhibition of IL-32 activation by alpha-1 antitrypsin suppresses alloreactivity and increases survival in an allogeneic murine marrow transplantation model. *Blood* , 118, 5031-5039.

[105] Marinkovic, S, et al. (1990). Structure, hormonal regulation, and identification of the interleukin-6- and dexamethasone-responsive element of the rat haptoglobin gene. *Mol Cell Biol* , 10, 1573-1583.

[106] Marquez, L, et al. (2012). Effects of haptoglobin polymorphisms and deficiency on susceptibility to inflammatory bowel disease and on severity of murine colitis. *Gut* , 61, 528-534.

[107] Martinez CorderoE, et al. ((2008). Alpha-1-acid glycoprotein, its local production and immunopathological participation in experimental pulmonary tuberculosis. *Tuberculosis (Edinb)* , 88, 203-211.

[108] Mashiba, S, et al. (2001). In vivo complex formation of oxidized alpha(1)-antitrypsin and LDL. *Arterioscler Thromb Vasc Biol* , 21, 1801-1808.

[109] Mejdoubi, N, et al. (1999). Growth hormone inhibits rat liver alpha-1-acid glycoprotein gene expression in vivo and in vitro. *Hepatology* , 29, 186-194.

[110] Mohanka, M, et al. (2012). A review of augmentation therapy for alpha-1 antitrypsin deficiency. *Expert Opin Biol Ther* , 12, 685-700.

[111] Montanelli, A, et al. (2002). Alpha-1-antitrypsin deficiency and nephropathy. *Nephron* , 90, 114-115.

[112] Muchitsch, E. M, et al. (1998). Effects of alpha 1-acid glycoprotein in different rodent models of shock. *Fundam Clin Pharmacol* , 12, 173-181.

[113] Muchitsch, E. M, et al. (1996). In vivo effect of alpha 1-acid glycoprotein on experimentally enhanced capillary permeability in guinea-pig skin. *Arch Int Pharmacodyn Ther* , 331, 313-321.

[114] Murakami, T, et al. (1993). Elevation of factor XIa-alpha 1-antitrypsin complex levels in NIDDM patients with diabetic nephropathy. *Diabetes* , 42, 233-238.

[115] Myles, D. A, et al. (1990). Rotation function studies of human C-reactive protein. *J Mol Biol* , 216, 491-496.

[116] Nakamura, T, et al. (1993). Alpha 1-acid glycoprotein expression in human leukocytes: possible correlation between alpha 1-acid glycoprotein and inflammatory cytokines in rheumatoid arthritis. *Inflammation* , 17, 33-45.

[117] Nevo, S. S, et al. (1968). Association between response to typhoid vaccination and known genetic markers. *Am J Hum Genet* , 20, 461-469.

[118] Ng, P. M, et al. (2007). C-reactive protein collaborates with plasma lectins to boost immune response against bacteria. *EMBO J* , 26, 3431-3440.

[119] Nita, I, et al. (2005). Prolastin, a pharmaceutical preparation of purified human alphaantitrypsin, blocks endotoxin-mediated cytokine release. *Respir Res* 6, 12., 1.

[120] Donoghue, O, et al. (1993). Alpha-1-proteinase inhibitor and pulmonary haemorrhage in systemic vasculitis. *Adv Exp Med Biol* , 336, 331-335.

[121] Riordan, O, et al. (1997). alpha 1-antitrypsin deficiency-associated panniculitis: resolution with intravenous alpha 1-antitrypsin administration and liver transplantation. *Transplantation* , 63, 480-482.

[122] Oh, S. K, et al. (1990). Specific binding of haptoglobin to human neutrophils and its functional consequences. *J Leukoc Biol* , 47, 142-148.

[123] Otterbein, L. E, et al. (2003). Heme oxygenase-1: unleashing the protective properties of heme. *Trends Immunol* , 24, 449-455.

[124] Ozeri, E, et al. (2012). alpha-1 antitrypsin promotes semimature, IL-10-producing and readily migrating tolerogenic dendritic cells. *J Immunol* , 189, 146-153.

[125] Paakko, P, et al. (1996). Activated neutrophils secrete stored alpha 1-antitrypsin. *Am J Respir Crit Care Med* , 154, 1829-1833.

[126] Parra, M. D, et al. (2006). Porcine acute phase protein concentrations in different diseases in field conditions. *J Vet Med B Infect Dis Vet Public Health* , 53, 488-493.

[127] Pepys, M. B, et al. (2003). C-reactive protein: a critical update. *J Clin Invest* , 111, 1805-1812.

[128] Perlmutter, D. H, et al. (1990). Endocytosis and degradation of alpha 1-antitrypsin-protease complexes is mediated by the serpin-enzyme complex (SEC) receptor. *J Biol Chem* , 265, 16713-16716.

[129] Perlmutter, D. H, et al. (1985). The cellular defect in alpha 1-proteinase inhibitor (alpha 1-PI) deficiency is expressed in human monocytes and in Xenopus oocytes injected with human liver mRNA. *Proc Natl Acad Sci U S A* , 82, 6918-6921.

[130] Perlmutter, D. H, et al. (1988). Distinct and additive effects of elastase and endotoxin on expression of alpha 1 proteinase inhibitor in mononuclear phagocytes. *J Biol Chem* , 263, 16499-16503.

[131] Perlmutter, D. H, et al. (1988). Elastase regulates the synthesis of its inhibitor, alpha 1-proteinase inhibitor, and exaggerates the defect in homozygous PiZZ alpha 1 PI deficiency. *J Clin Invest* , 81, 1774-1780.

[132] Petrache, I, et al. (2006). alpha-1 antitrypsin inhibits caspase-3 activity, preventing lung endothelial cell apoptosis. *Am J Pathol* , 169, 1155-1166.

[133] Piliang, M. P, et al. (2008). Women with ulcerating, painful skin lesions. *Cleve Clin J Med* 75, 414, 418, 422.

[134] Poller, W, et al. (1995). Differential recognition of alpha 1-antitrypsin-elastase and alpha 1-antichymotrypsin-cathepsin G complexes by the low density lipoprotein receptor-related protein. *J Biol Chem* , 270, 2841-2845.

[135] Poortmans, J, et al. (1968). Quantitative immunological determination of 12 plasma proteins excreted in human urine collected before and after exercise. *J Clin Invest* , 47, 386-393.

[136] Pos, O, et al. (1990). Con A-nonreactive human alpha 1-acid glycoprotein (AGP) is more effective in modulation of lymphocyte proliferation than Con A-reactive AGP serum variants. *Inflammation* , 14, 133-141.

[137] Potempa, L. A, et al. (1987). Expression, detection and assay of a neoantigen (Neo-CRP) associated with a free, human C-reactive protein subunit. *Mol Immunol* , 24, 531-541.

[138] Pries, A. R, et al. (2000). The endothelial surface layer. *Pflugers Arch* , 440, 653-666.

[139] Propst, T, et al. (1994). Alpha-1-antitrypsin deficiency and liver disease. *Dig Dis* , 12, 139-149.

[140] Rahman, M. M, et al. (2008). Alpha(1)-acid glycoprotein is contained in bovine neutrophil granules and released after activation. *Vet Immunol Immunopathol* , 125, 71-81.

[141] Ray, M. B, et al. (1982). Alpha-1-antitrypsin immunoreactivity in gastric carcinoid. *Histopathology* , 6, 289-297.

[142] Raynes, J. G, et al. (1991). Acute-phase protein synthesis in human hepatoma cells: differential regulation of serum amyloid A (SAA) and haptoglobin by interleukin-1 and interleukin-6. *Clin Exp Immunol* , 83, 488-491.

[143] Rees, R. F, et al. (1988). Expression of a C-reactive protein neoantigen (neo-CRP) in inflamed rabbit liver and muscle. *Clin Immunol Immunopathol* , 48, 95-107.

[144] Rossbacher, J, et al. (1999). Inhibitory effect of haptoglobin on granulocyte chemotaxis, phagocytosis and bactericidal activity. *Scand J Immunol* , 50, 399-404.

[145] Samak, R, et al. (1982). Immunosuppressive effect of acute-phase reactant proteins in vitro and its relevance to cancer. *Cancer Immunol Immunother* , 13, 38-43.

[146] Schaer, D. J, et al. (2006). CD163 is the macrophage scavenger receptor for native and chemically modified hemoglobins in the absence of haptoglobin. *Blood* , 107, 373-380.

[147] Schmid, K, et al. (1977). The carbohydrate units of human plasma alpha1-acid glycoprotein. *Biochim Biophys Acta* , 492, 291-302.

[148] Shin, S. Y, et al. (2011). Changes of Alpha1-Antitrypsin Levels in Allergen-induced Nasal Inflammation. *Clin Exp Otorhinolaryngol* , 4, 33-39.

[149] Shine, B, et al. (1981). Solid phase radioimmunoassays for human C-reactive protein. *Clin Chim Acta* , 117, 13-23.

[150] Siekmeier, R. (2010). Lung deposition of inhaled alpha-1-proteinase inhibitor (alpha 1-PI)- problems and experience of alpha1-PI inhalation therapy in patients with hereditary alpha1-PI deficiency and cystic fibrosis. *Eur J Med Res* 15 Suppl , 2, 164-174.

[151] Simons, K, et al. (2000). Lipid rafts and signal transduction. *Nat Rev Mol Cell Biol* , 1, 31-39.

[152] Sirica, A. E, et al. (1979). Fetal phenotypic expression by adult rat hepatocytes on collagen gel/nylon meshes. *Proc Natl Acad Sci U S A* , 76, 283-287.

[153] Slaughter, N, et al. (2003). The flotillins are integral membrane proteins in lipid rafts that contain TCR-associated signaling components: implications for T-cell activation. *Clin Immunol* , 108, 138-151.

[154] Smith, K. C, et al. (1989). Clinical and pathologic correlations in 96 patients with panniculitis, including 15 patients with deficient levels of alpha 1-antitrypsin. *J Am Acad Dermatol* , 21, 1192-1196.

[155] Smolarczyk, K, et al. (2005). Function-stabilizing mechanism of plasminogen activator inhibitor type 1 induced upon binding to alpha1-acid glycoprotein. *Biochemistry* , 44, 12384-12390.

[156] Sohrab, S, et al. (2009). Mechanism of alpha-1 antitrypsin endocytosis by lung endothelium. *FASEB J* , 23, 3149-3158.

[157] Sorensson, J, et al. (1999). Human endothelial cells produce orosomucoid, an important component of the capillary barrier. *Am J Physiol* 276, H, 530-534.

[158] Stockley, R. A, et al. (2010). Therapeutic efficacy of alpha-1 antitrypsin augmentation therapy on the loss of lung tissue: an integrated analysis of 2 randomised clinical trials using computed tomography densitometry. *Respir Res* 11, 136.

[159] Stocks, B. B, et al. (2012). Early Hydrophobic Collapse of alpha(1)-Antitrypsin Facilitates Formation of a Metastable State: Insights from Oxidative Labeling and Mass Spectrometry. *J Mol Biol*

[160] Su, S. J, et al. (1999). Alpha 1-acid glycoprotein-induced tumor necrosis factor-alpha secretion of human monocytes is enhanced by serum binding proteins and depends on protein tyrosine kinase activation. *Immunopharmacology* , 41, 21-29.

[161] Su, S. J, et al. (1996). Effects of alpha 1-acid glycoprotein on tissue factor expression and tumor necrosis factor secretion in human monocytes. *Immunopharmacology* , 34, 139-145.

[162] Subramaniyam, D, et al. (2006). C-36 peptide, a degradation product of alpha1-antitrypsin, modulates human monocyte activation through LPS signaling pathways. *Int J Biochem Cell Biol* , 38, 563-575.

[163] Subramaniyam, D, et al. (2008). TNF-alpha-induced self expression in human lung endothelial cells is inhibited by native and oxidized alpha1-antitrypsin. *Int J Biochem Cell Biol* , 40, 258-271.

[164] Subramaniyam, D, et al. (2010). Cholesterol rich lipid raft microdomains are gateway for acute phase protein, SERPINA1. *Int J Biochem Cell Biol* , 42, 1562-1570.

[165] Szalai, A. J, et al. (1995). Human C-reactive protein is protective against fatal Streptococcus pneumoniae infection in transgenic mice. *J Immunol* , 155, 2557-2563.

[166] Tawara, I, et al. (2012). Alpha-1-antitrypsin monotherapy reduces graft-versus-host disease after experimental allogeneic bone marrow transplantation. *Proc Natl Acad Sci U S A* , 109, 564-569.

[167] Taylor, K. E, et al. (2007). Structural and functional comparison of native pentameric, denatured monomeric and biotinylated C-reactive protein. *Immunology* , 120, 404-411.

[168] Theilgaard-monch, K, et al. (2005). Highly glycosylated alpha1-acid glycoprotein is synthesized in myelocytes, stored in secondary granules, and released by activated neutrophils. *J Leukoc Biol* , 78, 462-470.

[169] Tilg, H, et al. (1993). Antiinflammatory properties of hepatic acute phase proteins: preferential induction of interleukin 1 (IL-1) receptor antagonist over IL-1 beta synthesis by human peripheral blood mononuclear cells. *J Exp Med* , 178, 1629-1636.

[170] Tuder, R. M, et al. (2010). Lung disease associated with alpha1-antitrypsin deficiency. *Proc Am Thorac Soc* , 7, 381-386.

[171] Van Molle, W, et al. (1999). Activation of caspases in lethal experimental hepatitis and prevention by acute phase proteins. *J Immunol* , 163, 5235-5241.

[172] Vigushin, D. M, et al. (1993). Metabolic and scintigraphic studies of radioiodinated human C-reactive protein in health and disease. *J Clin Invest* , 91, 1351-1357.

[173] Volanakis, J. E, et al. (1981). Interaction of C-reactive protein with artificial phosphatidylcholine bilayers and complement. *J Immunol* , 126, 1820-1825.

[174] Wagner, L, et al. (1996). Haptoglobin phenotyping by newly developed monoclonal antibodies. Demonstration of haptoglobin uptake into peripheral blood neutrophils and monocytes. *J Immunol* , 156, 1989-1996.

[175] Warnock, D. E, et al. (1993). Determination of plasma membrane lipid mass and composition in cultured Chinese hamster ovary cells using high gradient magnetic affinity chromatography. *J Biol Chem* , 268, 10145-10153.

[176] Weinhold, B, et al. (1997). Interleukin-6 is necessary, but not sufficient, for induction of the humanC-reactive protein gene in vivo. *Biochem J* 325 (Pt 3), 617-621.

[177] Wiemer, A. J, et al. (2010). Calpain inhibition impairs TNF-alpha-mediated neutrophil adhesion, arrest and oxidative burst. *Mol Immunol* , 47, 894-902.

[178] Wu, L, et al. (2005). The low-density lipoprotein receptor-related protein-1 associates transiently with lipid rafts. *J Cell Biochem* , 96, 1021-1033.

[179] Yoon, I. S, et al. (2007). Low-density lipoprotein receptor-related protein promotes amyloid precursor protein trafficking to lipid rafts in the endocytic pathway. *FASEB J* , 21, 2742-2752.

[180] Yoshioka, M, et al. (2002). Regulation of haptoglobin secretion by recombinant bovine cytokines in primary cultured bovine hepatocytes. *Domest Anim Endocrinol* , 23, 425-433.

[181] Yu, S. J, et al. (1999). Attenuation of haptoglobin gene expression by TGFbeta requires the MAP kinase pathway. *Biochem Biophys Res Commun* , 259, 544-549.

[182] Zhang, B, et al. (2007). Alpha1-antitrypsin protects beta-cells from apoptosis. *Diabetes* , 56, 1316-1323.

[183] Zhang, D, et al. (1995). The effect of interleukin-1 on C-reactive protein expression in Hep3B cells is exerted at the transcriptional level. *Biochem J* 310 (Pt 1), 143-148.

[184] Zhang, J, et al. (2009). Local inflammation induces complement crosstalk which amplifies the antimicrobial response. *PLoS Pathog* 5, e1000282.

[185] Zhu, D, et al. (2006). Lipid rafts serve as a signaling platform for nicotinic acetylcholine receptor clustering. *J Neurosci* , 26, 4841-4851.

[186] Zouki, C, et al. (1997). Prevention of In vitro neutrophil adhesion to endothelial cells through shedding of L-selectin by C-reactive protein and peptides derived from C-reactive protein. *J Clin Invest* , 100, 522-529.

[187] Zouki, C, et al. (2001). Loss of pentameric symmetry of C-reactive protein is associated with promotion of neutrophil-endothelial cell adhesion. *J Immunol* , 167, 5355-5361.

Chapter 2

Inflammation and Acute Phase Proteins in Haemostasis

Simon J. Davidson

Additional information is available at the end of the chapter

http://dx.doi.org/10.5772/55998

1. Introduction

Inflammation is a very complex reaction to infection or injury the endeavour being to contain the infection and harm to a limited area. The process is associated with the activation of the coagulation system. To think that inflammation occurs and then leads to activation of the coagulation system is not quite true as there is much cross-talk between the two systems. This is a natural host response to cellular damage or infection however an overshooting of this cross-talk between coagulation and inflammation can lead to an exaggerated prothrombotic state and exacerbate the disease process. A wide range of inflammatory conditions such as infections, acute respiratory distress syndrome and SIRS (systemic inflammatory response syndrome) following major surgery e.g.cardiac surgery can lead to an uncontrolled inflammatory response and to profound disturbance of the coagulation system leading to an imbalance in the normal anticoagulated state of blood to that of a procoagulant state. When coagulation is compromised it can contribute to the pathogenesis of the inflammatory condition with deposition of fibrin within the microvasculature directly enhancing the inflammatory reaction. This in turn leads to a modulation of protein manufacture mainly via Liver hepatocytes in the upregulation and downregulation of at least twenty factors directly involved in blood coagulation. This process is controlled via cytokines and leads to the imbalance in what are called the haemostatic acute phase proteins. All of which puts the haemostatic system at an increased thrombotic potential [1, 2, 3, 4].

The haemostatic system maintains blood in a fluid phase under normal physiological conditions and provides a mechanism to prevent exsanguination upon vascular damage. Morawitz had created the 'classic' theory of blood coagulation in 1905 but it was Macfarlane who first reported the coagulation cascade as a biochemical amplification pathway of pro-enzyme-enzyme transformations in 1964 [5]. Davie and Ratnoff later the same year referred to it as a waterfall stepwise sequence of activation [6]. Macfarlane's idea that amplification of the cascade and acceleration of earlier stages of the pathway culminating in the conversion of fibrinogen to fibrin was a major breakthrough in the understanding of how the coagulation factors interacted and forms the basis of what we understand today.

Platelets are the primary haemostatic plug when damage first occurs to a vessel. The multimeric protein von Willebrand factor mediates the adhesion of platelets to the site of vascular damage. The platelets bind to the matrix proteins exposed by the damage to the vessel wall, particularly collagen. These platelets are activated by small amounts of thrombin (~1nM) produced by tissue factor exposure at the site of vascular damage. The tissue factor binds factor VII that is rapidly activated. The tissue factor-VIIa complex subsequently activates factor X. The activated platelet provides binding sites for the coagulation enzymes, localising coagulation to the site of injury and prolonging activation of coagulation by protecting the enzymes from inhibition and inactivation [7]. Factor X is essential to this 'propagation' phase of coagulation. When bound to the platelet and activated via the VIIIa-IXa complex Xa is protected from inhibition by tissue factor pathway inhibitor and antithrombin.

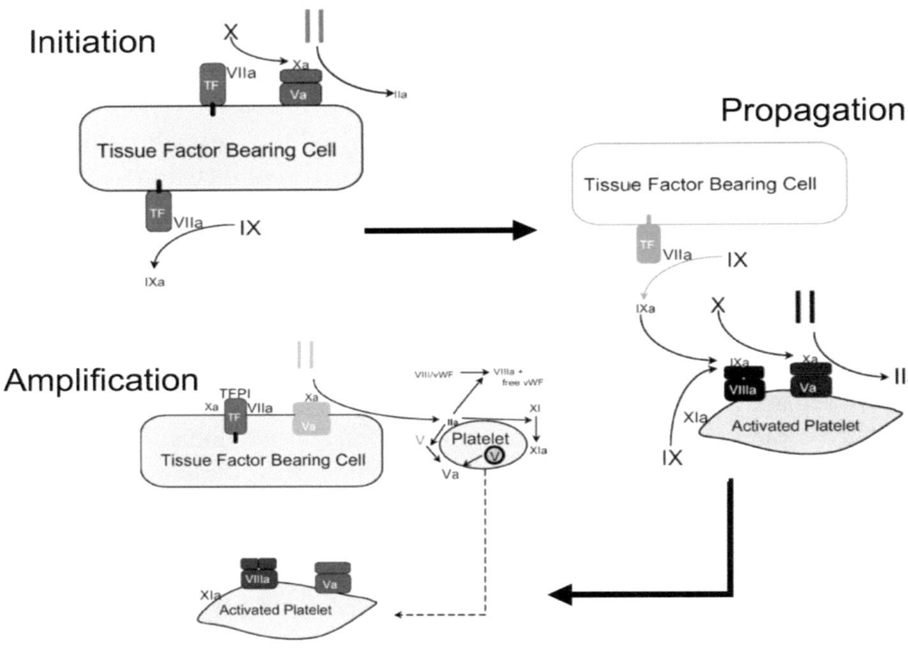

Figure 1. Cell based model coagulation. Reproduced with kind permission of Professor M.Hoffman

Tissue factor pathway inhibitor (TFPI) rapidly blunts this driving force of tissue factor-VIIa complex that initiates coagulation and generates the sudden burst of thrombin [8]. Once trace amounts of thrombin have been formed this is then able to activate factors V, VIII, IX and XI. This positive feedback mechanism ensures prolonged activation of the system with sufficient quantities of thrombin being produced to activate platelets, white cells, endothelial cells, and the protein C anticoagulant pathway and to continue producing thrombin.

http://dx.doi.org/10.5772/55998

Coagulation activation yields proteases that not only interact with coagulation protein zymogens but also with specific cell receptors to induce signaling pathways that mediate inflammatory responses [9]. Many in vitro observations point to a role of coagulation proteases in upregulating the expression of proinflammatory mediators [10]. The most important mechanism by which coagulation proteases influence inflammation is by binding to protease activated receptors (PARs), of which four types (PAR 1 to 4) have been identified, all belonging to the family of transmembrane domain, G-protein–coupled receptors [11]. Tissue factor is also a potential mediator of intracellular signaling of established inflammatory pathways, functioning as an intermediate for factor VIIa–induced activation of mitogen-activated protein kinases and calcium signalling [12]. It is tissue factor that binds to factor VII and drives thrombin generation leading to fibrin formation. Tissue factor is an integral membrane protein normally separated from blood by the vascular endothelium. Tissue factor is expressed in the vascular adventitia in astroglial cells. It also appears in tumour cells where it appears related to their metastatic potential. All of this activation of coagulation increases in some procoagulant factors (fibrinogen and fator VIII) with reduced fibrinolytic response and dampening of the natural anticoagulant potential have a profound effect on mortality.

Thrombin plays many parts (Figure 2) and with the anticoagulant protein, activated protein C, can activate specific cell receptors on mononuclear cells and endothelial cells which can affect cytokine production and inflammatory cell apoptosis.

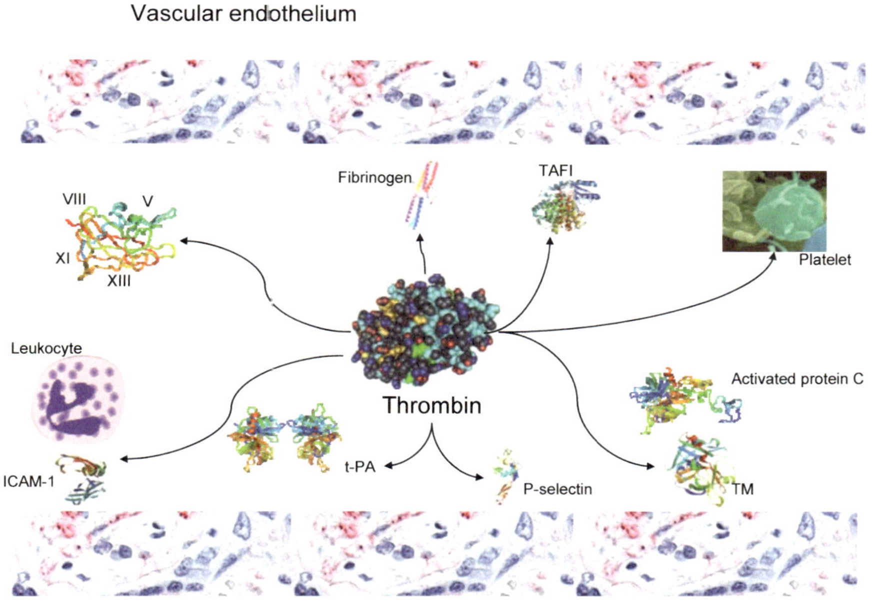

Figure 2. Thrombins role in activating scme of the components of coagulation and inflammation. Coagulation factors V, VIII,XI and XIII, TM – thrombomodulin, TAFI – thrombin activatable fibrinolytic inhibitor, t-PA – tissue plasminogen activator, ICAM-1 intracellular adhesion molecule 1

2. Initiation of the pro-inflammatory response

Pathogen recognition receptors, Toll receptors (TLR), are essential in the host defence against pathogens. Platelets express these pattern recognition receptors involved in innate immunity. TLR's recognise microbial structures that are conserved among species. TLR1,2,4 6,8 & 9 all appear on platelets and form one of the many bridges between inflammation and coagulation. TLR's are responsible for LPS induced thrombocytopenia [13]. Platelets express TLR – pattern recognition receptors involved in innate immunity. TLR's are able to recognise danger associated molecular patterns (DAMPs). For example fibrinogen that is released during inflammation is a DAMP and further enhances the proinflammatory response through TLR4. It is via TLR and DAMPs that induction of caspase-1 activation which causes the processing of the proinflammatory response through various cytokines [14]. Figure 3

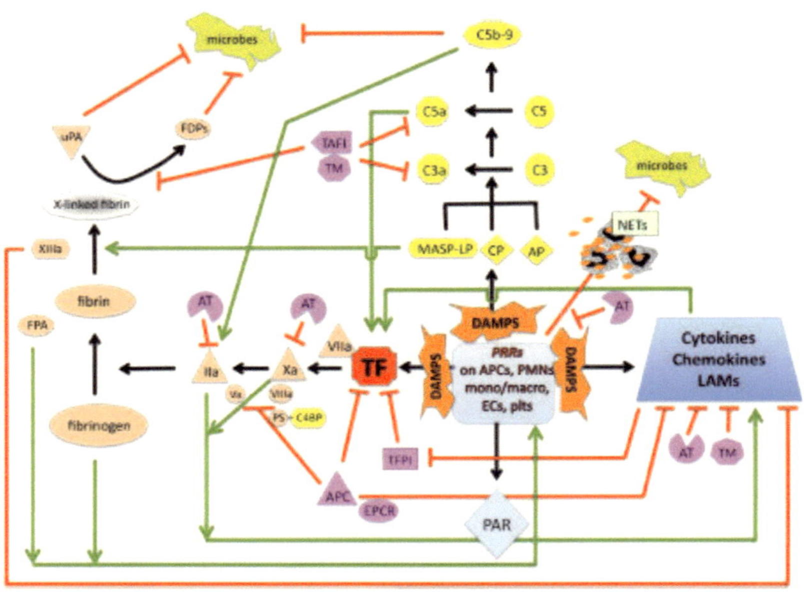

Figure 3. Cross-talk between coagulation and innate immune pathways in response to DAMPs (danger associated molecular patterns); DAMPS from invading pathogens or damaged host cellsare recognised by pathogen recognition receptors (PRRs) on antigen presenting cells, neutrophils, monocytes, macropahges, endothelial cells and platelets. This results in tissue factor exposure sustained by cytokines and chemokines with proinflammatory and opsonic properties and associated with increaased expressionof leukocyte adhesion molecules. In parallel DAMP-induced complement activation via any of the complement activation pathways leads to generation of the complement factors C3a and C5a and the membrane attack complex C5b-9. C5a feeds back to promote further tissue factor expresssion and C5b-9 also supports generation of thrombin. Green lines indicate increase n response, red lines indicate supression. Reproduced with kind permission of Dr EM Conway.

Cytokines are small molecules that have relatively short half-lives of between minutes and hours but play a pivotal role in the inflammatory response. The most important cytokines

http://dx.doi.org/10.5772/55998

involved in regulating the coagulation response during inflammation are IL-6, TNF-alpha, IL-8, MCP-1 and IL-1 [15].

Acute phase proteins are released as mediators of the inflammatory cascade as a chemical and cellular response to injury. They increase rapidly in plasma in response to a inflammatory insult. Some acute phase proteins increase transiently (C-reactive protein) while others have a more sustained elevation (Haptoglobin) [16].

The inflammatory response to surgery, atherosclerosis, infection and cardiovascular disease has a profound effect upon the haemostatic system, including fibrinolysis. The cytokines interleukin 1β (IL-1β) and interleukin 6 (IL-6) modulate the production and suppression of many of the coagulation enzymes formed by the Liver.

The effect is to make the endothelium and whole coagulation system more procoagulant. Figure 4

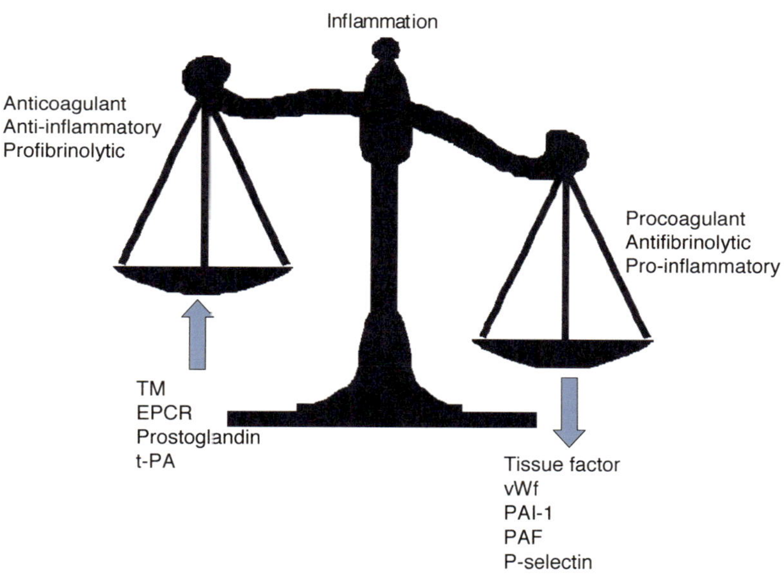

Figure 4. Inflammatory drive to a procoagulant state following endothelial stimulation.

3. Coagulation acute phase proteins

An acute-phase protein has been defined as one whose plasma concentration increases (positive acute-phase proteins) or decreases (negative acute-phase proteins) by at least 25 percent during inflammatory disorders [16]. The changes in the concentrations of acute-phase proteins are due largely to changes in their production by hepatocytes. Although the mechanism by which the liver processes the stimulation to increase and decrease protein production may be different in different forms of inflammatory insult e.g. sepsis and chronic inflammation [17].

Proteins whose plasma concentrations increase with inflammation	Proteins whose plasma concentrations decrease with inflammation
Fibrinogen	Factor XII
Factor VIII	Antithrombin
Protein S	Histidine rich glycoprotein
Plasminogen activator inhibitor PAI-1 C4b-binding	Thrombomodulin
protein	Endothelial protein C receptor
Urokinase	Thrombin activatable fibrinolytic inhibitor TAFI?
α 1 Antitrypsin	Protein C (? No change/decrease)
α 2 Macrogloulin	
von Willebrand factor	
C1-esterase inhibitor	
C-reactive protein	
Thrombopoietin	
Thrombin activatable fibrinolytic inhibitor (TAFI)?	

Table 1. Acute phase proteins that directly affect haemostasis

4. Coagulation proteins whose plasma concentrations increase during inflammation

4.1. Fibrinogen

Fibrinogen is a soluble glycoprotein synthesised in the Liver with a normal plasma concentration of 2 – 4 g/L and half life of 4 days. When the coagulation cascade is activated fibrinogen is the final substrate in the formation of a clot being converted to its insoluble fibrin form. Thrombin cleaves fibrinogen releasing fibrinopeptide A and B forming fibrin monomers which have exposed polymerisation sites on the fibrin molecule. Thrombin activates factor XIII which cross-links these fibrin fibrils increasing clot strength and rendering them more resistant to proteolysis [18]. Fibrin creation is required with platelets (stimulating platelet aggregation by binding to the glycoprotein IIb/IIIa platelet membrane receptor) to repair any breach in the vascular integrity and prevent haemorrhage. This process is not left unchecked and is regulated via the fibrinolytic system (plasmin production) to prevent excess fibrin accumulation at the site of damage despite the procoagulant signalling drive. The local production of plasmin is regulated via two plasminogen activators, tissue plasminogen activator (t-PA) and urokinase plasminogen activator (u-PA) which under normal physiological conditions keeps this fibrin matrix production and its lysis tightly controlled [19].

http://dx.doi.org/10.5772/55998

During an inflammatory reaction fibrinogen can increase in the order of 2-3 fold and this will significantly increase blood viscosity and cause some degree of red cell aggregation as well as transform vascular pathologies such as atherosclerotic plaques. Fibrinogen by means of increasing the production of endothelin-1, is also capable of directly inducing vasoconstriction [18].

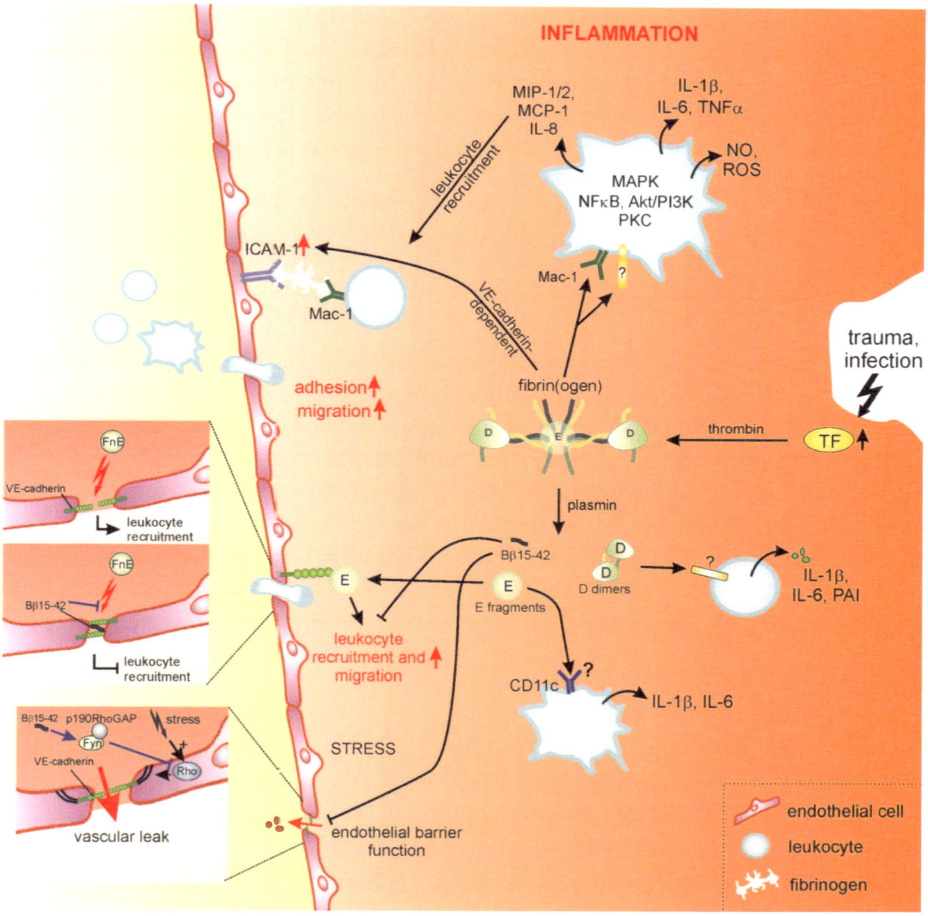

Figure 5. Fibrinogen and fibrin modulation of inflammation. Fibrin(ogen) modulates the inflammatory response by affecting leukocyte migration but also by induction of cytokine/chemokine expression mostly via Mac-1 signalling. NO-nitric oxide, Mac-1 Macrophage antigen 1, PI3K Phosphoinositide-3-kiniase, TNF tumor necrosis factor. Reproduced with kind permission of Prof. K Zacharowski

There is good evidence that fibrinogen has a function in regulation of the inflammatory response as is seen in the increased concentration of fibrinogen associated with atherosclerosis and cardiovascular risk. Fibrin(ogen) also participates in activation of vascular cells and regulation of the inflammatory response via the ability to bind to and activate a number of immune cells. The cellular ligand binding of fibrinogen is totally distinct to any coagulation function. Fibrin(ogen) can bind to the integrin receptor Mac-1 which is found on many myeloid cells including monocytes and neutrophils and also T cells. The Mac-1 integrin is involved in phagocytosis, adhesion, migration through the endothelium as well as apoptosis and degranulation (Figure 5). Binding of fibrinogen to Mac-1 also induces production of cytokines IL-1β, IL-6 and TNF-α potentiating the inflammatory response, as many acute phase proteins do [20].

When fibrin is laid down in the microvasculature bed this enhances local and systemic inflammation via expression of proinflammatory mediators. Fibrin(ogen) increases mRNA concentration and induces synthesis of the proinflammatory cytokines IL-6 and TNF-α in monocytes and macrophages which is induced by chemokine expression, macrophage chemotactic protein (MCP-1) and macrophage inflammatory protein (MIP-1 and 2). The Toll receptor TLR 4 facilitates this fibrin(gen) chemokine expression signalling [20].

Breakdown products of fibrin, D-dimers stimulate monocytes to release the following IL-1, IL-6 and PAI-1 and fibrin degradation products also induce C-reactive protein production.

4.2. Factor VIII

Factor VIII is a procoagulant whose deficiency leads to classical haemophilia and a bleeding diathesis [21]. Factor VIII once activated by small amounts of thrombin becomes a co-factor for activated factor IXa in the formation of the tenase complex whereby these catalysts convert factor X to its activated form Xa. A number of publications have shown raised factor VIII to be linked with venous thromboembolism and increased thrombin generation [22, 23]. This increase in factor VIII has been linked with an increase in basal inflammatory reaction. Factor VIII increased production is mediated by the cytokine IL-6, however it is debateable as to how much a persistently raised factor VIII is responsible to inflammation by some [24]. Post operatively particularly after cardiac surgery factor VIII can be raised by as much as 2-3 fold.

4.3. Protein S

Protein S is a co-factor for protein C and produced mainly in the hepatocyes but also endothelial cells and megakaryocytes. Once protein C has been activated by the thrombin thrombomodulin complex, which is augmented by the endothelial protein C receptor, activated protein C dissociates from the endothelial protein C receptor and binds with protein S. This complex is then able to inhibit factors Va and VIIIa, protein S enhancing the reactive cleaving of specific sites by APC on factors V and VIII by anything up to 20-fold. At any one time only approximately 40% of circulating protein S is free and able to participate in this reaction. The remaining 60% of circulating protein S is bound to the complement regulator protein C4B-binding protein and lacks the co-factor functionality in this reaction. Consequently the protein S-C4BP complex limits the functionality of activated protein C in its anticoagulant role. Therefore protein S plays an important role in the regulation of thrombin generation although it being a risk factor for venous thrombosis in deficient patients remains unclear and the odds risks have varied between 0 – 11.5 fold in protein S deficient cases.

Protein S has an accelerating role in APC mediated PAI-1 inhibition thereby promoting clot lysis and a possible inhibition of activation of thrombin activatable fibrinolytic inhibitor [25].

Protein S has been shown to increase during inflammation. This may in part be due to counterbalancing the procoagulant drive of the coagulation system in these circumstances by providing more anticoagulant effect via the protein C pathway. It may also have to do with other non-anticoagulant actions it has via its binding with C4BP (see below). Certainly inhibition of protein S in in-vivo models of bacteraemia have shown to provoke the cytokine response and what was a non-lethal injected dose of *E.coli* in baboons resulted in a lethal reaction [26].

4.4. C4b-binding protein

The complement binding protein C4BP is a co-factor to a serine protease in the degradation of C4 in the classical complement pathway and providing it has been suggested protection from inflammation at a cellular level. The C4BP molecule has a central region with seven α chains and one β chain emanating from it each with distinct ligand binding regions. It is on the β chain side arm that the protein S binding region resides and in normal human plasma ~80% of C4BP is found as this β chain form. C4BP is an acute phase protein and its levels can increase to 400% of normal [25]. However this is mainly of the C4BPα form so the Protein S-C4BP complex concentration is not generally affected. As so much protein S is normally bound to C4BP and the concentration of the free anticoagulant active co-factor protein S level quite tightly controlled is there a physiological role for the PS-C4BP complex? It has been suggested that protein S forms one of the bridges between coagulation and inflammation. As protein S has a high affinity to bind to negatively charged phospholipids it can bring C4BP into close proximity to these sites allowing controlled complement activation at areas of vascular damage where coagulation is activated. This has been linked to apoptosis and the complement system allowing rapid clearance of apoptotic cells from the site of damage by macrophages but more probably limiting or inhibiting further complement activation via necrotic cells [27, 28].

4.5. Plasminogen activator inhibitor PAI-1

The fibrinolytic system is the opposite of the coagulation system. It limits clot formation to the site of injury and breaks down existing clot by an enzyme cascade. It is also, like haemostasis, linked to inflammation with acute phase proteins that increase and others that are decreased. Plasminogen provides the fibrinolytic potential and when converted to its active form plasmin is able to bind to fibrin and begin its degradation. Plasminogen is activated by two activators, tissue plasminogen activator (t-PA) and urokinase tissue plasmingen activator (u-PA). These in turn are inhibited by plasminogen activator inhibitor 1 and 2 (PAI-1, PAI-2) and plasmin is inhibited by α-2-antiplasmin. Of these inhibitors PAI-1 is a positive acute phase protein and increases during inflammation. The cytokine tissue necrosis factor

(TNF-α) suppresses finbrinolysis by down regulating t-PA expression in endothelial cells while production PAI-1 then in turn PAI-1 inhibits TNF-α is inhibited by PAI-1. It has also been shown that by inhibiting TNF-α plasma levels of PAI-1 decrease [19].

The increase in PAI-1 levels is again a driver of the haemostatic system towards a more prothrombotic state. PAI-2 will not be discussed here but for interested readers they are directed to the following publication [29].

4.6. Urokinase

Urokinase plasminogen activator (u-PA) is a multifunctional serine protease. It has been shown to act as both a signalling ligand and a proteolytic enzyme. As an acute phase protein its increase has been found in a number of metastatic carcinomas and this has led to a link in its role of tumor growth and cellular expansion in conditions such as cardiac fibrosis and atherosclerosis [30]. As well as displaying involvement in tissue remodelling u-PA also appears to regulate macrophage activation and function. The macrophages not only synthesis and release u-PA but also have receptors for the u-PA protease on their membranes. The excreted u-PA induces TNF-α synthesis and secretion. The u-PA molecule has also been shown to initiate inflammation via the release of IL-6 and IL-1β from monocytes and lymphocytes [31]. The u-PA and its receptor uPAR also mediate immune complex induced inflammation in the lung. This is achieved via generation of u-PA at the site of cellular inflammation with subsequent activation of its receptor uPAR. This then sets off cellular signalling with C5a/C5aR on the alveolar macrophages, recruitment of polymorphonuclear leukocytes and adequate TNF-α production [32].

4.7. α 1 Antitrypsin

The α-1-antitrypsin glycoprotein is a proteinase inhibitor synthesised and secreted in the hepatocytes of the Liver. It is one of two physiological inhibtors of activated protein C. It also has a profound anti-inflammatory effect in the lungs with concentrations during a inflammatory response reaching levels found in the plasma. The range of antiprotease activity seen in the lungs includes neutrophil elastase and plasminogen acitvators. If there is a deficiency of α-1-antitrypsin (as with the genetically abnormal SERPINA1 gene mutations) then neutrophil elastase provoked by infection and inflammation will unchecked breakdown elastin and destroy alveolar walls leading to emphysema [33].

4.8. Alpha-2-macroglobulin

Alpha-2-Macroglobulin (α-2M) is an ancient serine protease binding host or foreign peptides and particles, thereby serving as humoral defense barrier against pathogens in the plasma and tissues. In humans α-2M, interacts and captures virtually any proteinase whether self or foreign, suggesting a function as a unique "panproteinase inhibitor." In adult humans it provides somewhere between 10-25% of the overall anti-thrombin activity in plasma. It is also the primary inhibitor of thrombin in neonates and infants under 1 year of age until the Liver matures and begins producing sufficient Antithrombin to take over the role. At times of inflammation when antithrombin levels are low α-2M can become a 'back-up' thrombin inhibitor [34].

4.9. C1-esterase inhibitor

C1-inhibitor (C1INH) is a serpin and major inhibitor of the contact coagulation system that involves factor XII, kallikrein and kininogen. It is also an important regulator of complement activation inhibiting the first component of complement C1. Another important biological role of C1INH is vascular permeability regulation [35]. This is well illustrated in patients who suffer from hereditary angioedema where there is a deficiency of the C1INH activity. As it now seems factor XII plays a substantial part in the formation of thrombin during sepsis and inflammation where neutrophil extracellular traps are present that release polyphosphate that in turn activate factor XII it would appear normal for C1INH to act as a positive acute phase protein in limiting this activation as well as its complement inhibitory role. A rapid appearance of C1INH-factor XIIa complexes is reported during sepsis with a sharp fall in the C1INH activity wherein the inhibitory function of α-2Macroglobin becomes more important in its kallikrein inhibiting role [36].

4.10. von Willebrand factor

The von Willebrand factor (VWF) is a multimeric protein that mediates the adhesion of platelets to the exposed subendothelium at the site of vascular injury. It also serves as a carrier protein for the labile coagulation factor VIII. VWF is synthesised in and stored in the Weibal-Palade bodies of endothelial cells and megakaryocytes/platelets. Endothelial cells release VWF when activated or stimulated. These VWF molecules are ultralarge and hyperactive, proficient in binding to platelets via the glycoprotein Ib-X-V complex without any external activation. Normally the ultralarge VWF multimers are cleaved into smaller less active multimers before being released into plasma. Cleavage is performed by ADAMTS-13 (a disintegrin and metalloprotease with thrombospondin motif). A deficiency of ADAMTS-13 leads to a thrombotic thrombocytopenic purpura a thrombotic microangiopathy. Increased plasma levels of VWF have been reported in a number of disease states including coronary artery disease, autoimmune disease, trauma and infections. A common underlying process in all of these is inflammation. There appears to be a complex interaction between the common inflammatory cytokines IL-6, IL-1β and TNF-α the release and cleavage of the VWF multimers by ADAMTS-13.

Release of VWF multimers from endothelial cells occurs in a dose dependent fashion when stimulated with IL-8 and TNF-α and IL-6 inhibits cleavage of the ultrlarge multimers. This demonstrates that inflammatory cytokines interfere with the equilibrium of release and rate of cleavage of the ultralarge VWF multimers.

This increases prothrombotic risk in this setting as most of the positive acute phase proteins have a propensity to do creating a procoagulant environment. It is of interest to note that IL-8 resides in the Weibel-Palade bodies of the platelet the same place as VWF and is involved in the platelet leukocyte aggregation and it is TNF-α that activates endothelial cells releasing IL-8. The inhibition by IL-6 of ultralarge multimer cleavage by ADAMTS-13 may be by way of synthetic and secretion inhibition. In overwhelming sepsis there is also probably an element of exhaustion of metalloprotease activity [37].

4.11. C-reactive protein

C-reactive protein (CRP) is a pentameric molecule that increases several hundred fold following an inflammatory stimulatory response this being primarily due to IL-6 stimulation of production of CRP in the hepatocytes of the Liver. CRP amplifies the host defence mechanism by activation of complement via C1 and stimulation of macrophages. CRP also upregulates tissue factor expression on monocytes [38] and induces release of PAI-1 thereby downregulating fibrinolysis [39] promoting a procoagulant state. The pentameric CRP is thought to be directly proinflammatory at high concentration like those of sepsis or major surgery but more subtle inflammatory reactions take place when monomeric CRP is released from the pentameric form. This appears to be driven by activated platelets revealing new lipid messenger sites; lysophosphatidycholine (LPC) that bind and dissociate the pentameric form of CRP to the monmeric form [40].

During sepsis when disseminated intravascular coagulation (DIC) occurs this has been found experimentally to co-inside with formation of a calcium-dependent complex between CRP and very low density lipoprotein (VLDL). The VLDL molecular makeup is different in septic patients to normal controls due to a deficiency of phosphatidylethanolamine. This CRP-VLDL lipid raft increases the procoagulant effect through an increase in prothrombinase activity. The CRP-VLDL complex exists in vivo and it has been postulated that is has a pathogenic role in disseminating the intravascular coagulation [41].

5. Coagulation proteins whose plasma concentrations decrease during inflammation

5.1. Antithrombin

Antithrombin (AT) is one of the major natural anticoagulats inhibiting thrombin, factor Xa, IXa and factor VIIa bound to tissue factor. Inhibition of factors Xa, IXa and the VIIa-tissue factor are accelerated via the endothelial cell heparin like proteoglycans. The importance of this anticoagulant pathway is highlighted when AT levels are low, either congenitally or acquired, the risk of thrombosis is significantly increased.

AT has been shown in-vitro using HUVEC cells and IL-6 to act as a negative acute phase protein [42]. Other mechanisms that can reduce AT function during an inflammatory response include increased consumption from activation of haemostasis and increased degradation by proteolytic enzymes (elastase released from activated neutrophils). Furthermore inflammatory cytokines can induce a reduction in the production of glycosaminoglycans such as heparin and chondroitin sulphate on the endothelial cell which may contribute to the impaired function of AT due to GAGs acting as physiological heparin-like cofactors promoting the anticoagulant anti-thrombin activity of AT [43, 44].

AT can indirectly act as an anti-inflammatory molecule by directly inhibiting thrombin reducing its inflammatory properties of haemostatic and complement activation, leukocyte, endothelial and platelet activation. AT also appears to directly act as an anti-inflammatory agent by binding with leukocytes receptors blocking their communication with endothelial cells and limiting their adhesion and migration [45]. In animal models it has also been shown that AT induces the release of prostacyclin from endothelial cells. The prostacyclin is a platelet inhibitor and abrogates neutrophils adhering to endothelial cells both of which contribute to the inflammatory response [46].

In addition AT can also modulate cellular receptor expression by downregulating the expression of CD11b/CD18 on leucocytes which bind factor X aiding its activation [47].

AT is also able to decrease expression of tissue factor and IL-6 expression on monocytes and endothelial cells reducing the inflammatory drive [48].

5.2. Histidine rich glycoprotein

Histindine rich glycoprotein (HRGP) is a single polypeptide chain protein that is synthesised in the Liver found in plasma and on the surface of leukocytes, monocytes and the α-granules of platelets. HRGP has been shown to bind to a number of molecules including, haem, Zn^{2+}, plasminogen, fibrinogen, IgG, complement and factor XIIa (not the inactive zymogen) [49]. HRGP exerts some degree of innate immune response by exhibiting antimicrobial activity to some organisms and removal of necrotic cells by binding to free decondensed DNA (polyphosphate).

HRGP behaves as a negative acute protein during inflammation [50]. This is of interest as fibrinogen one of its primary ligands is increased. Possibly more importantly is the fact that HRGP strongly inhibits polyphosphate induced factor XII autoactivation via increased Zn^{2+} levels in response to local platelet activation, showing it to be a significant modulator of factor XII activation during sepsis and inflammation [51]. Because of its negative acute phase nature this will allow increased activation of factor XII in these circumstances potentiating the pro-inflammatory and pro-coagulant condition.

5.3. Thrombomodulin

Thrombomodulin (TM) is present on endothelial cells of the entire vasculature and is a transmembrane protein with epidermal growth factor (EGF) repeating molecules that stick out of the plasma membrane and provide binding and activation sites for a number of molecules. There is a high affinity binding site for thrombin on EGF domain 5-6 from which protein C is activated at EGF domains 4-6. Thrombin activatable fibrinolytic inhibitor is activated by thrombin at EGF sites 3-6 [52]. When thrombin binds and complexes with thrombomodulin on the cell membrane its ability to activate protein C increases by greater than 1000-fold. Activated protein C anti-inflammatory effects are discussed later in this chapter, see below. Once thrombin has bound to TM it becomes quickly neutralised by its natural serine proteases inhibitors antithrombin, heparin co-factor II and protein C inhibitor and therefore activation of protein C also ceases.

The effect of inflammation on TM is to decrease its presence on the endothelial cell surface by its cellular internalisation by endocytosis via TNF-α. This creates a site where coagulation can take place as the anticoagulant barrier has been removed and it may also stimulated further inflammatory response [43]. CRP has also been shown in experimental conditions using human coronary artery endothelial cells treated with CRP in a dose and time dependent manner to reduce messenger RNA levels of TM [53]. TM also provides anti-inflammatory protection from complement activation by enhancing inactivation of C3b and by promoting activation of thrombin-activatable fibrinolysis inhibitor that inactivates complement anaphylatoxins C5a and C3a [54]. Others have shown that thrombin-activatable fibrinolysis inhibitor activation via TM is attenuated by platelet factor 4 released from activated platelets [55].

5.4. Endothelial protein C receptor

The thrombomodulin-thrombin conversion of protein C to its activated form is facilitated by the endothelial protein C receptor (EPCR). The EPCR is another endothelial cell transmembrane protein located in close proximity to the thrombomodulin molecule and with high affinity binding for protein C. EPCR as well as binding protein C also binds its activated form and via membrane lipid rafts they complex with PAR-1 [56]. The EPCR-activated protein C molecule activates PAR-1 in a different way to thrombin which allows it to signal through a potent Gi protein pathway by which anti-inflammatory pathways are stimulated within the endothelial cell [57]. C-reactive protein has also been shown, as in the case of thrombomodulin, under experimental cell culture conditions to down regulate EPCR.

5.5. Thrombin activatable fibrinolytic inhibitor

Thrombin activatable fibrinolytic inhibitor (TAFI) is a basic carboxypeptidase identical to the plasma procarboxypeptidases B, U and R. TAFI is activated by thrombin and plasmin although the most efficient activator is the thrombomodulin-thrombin cellular membrane bound complex. TAFI inhibits fibrinolysis by cleaving lysine residues from fibrin which restricts the binding of tissue plasminogen activator to these sites and enhancing the plasminogen conversion to plasmin potentiating further fibrin breakdown [58]. TAFI certainly modulates the balance between coagulation and fibrinolysis but it appears its linking role with inflammation still needs to be fully elucidated. For instance TAFI has been shown to be a positive acute phase protein in mice [59] but in the same year Boffa et al interestingly showed that IL-6 administered to cultured HepG2 cells resulted in a 60% decrease in TAFI mRNA [58]. Subsequently TAFI has been shown to be raised in experimental endotoxemia [60]. Its anti-inflammatory properties are also downregulated by platelet factor 4 which is release from activated platelets and endothelial cells during activating stimuli and inflammatory insults which prevents TAFI activation by binding to the thrombin-thrombomodulin complex thereby preventing TAFI's inactivation of the complement anaphylatoxins C5a and C3a [55].

http://dx.doi.org/10.5772/55998

6. Other major components of the acute phase response that affect haemostasis

6.1. Protein C

The protein C pathway is known to be an important anticoagulant system with patients deficient in protein C being at risk of thrombosis or in its homozygous form purpura fulminans. Activated protein C inhibits factors V and VIII this being supported by the activation of protein C by thrombin bound to thrombomodulin on the endothelial cell surface. As well as acting as an anticoagulant activated protein C is also able to inhibit PAI-1. The anticoagulant and antifibrinolytic aspects of the protein C pathway have been elucidated and well described although there still appears much to learn from the interaction of protein C during the inflammatory response.

It is unclear from studies of the acute phase proteins whether protein C acts as a positive or negative acute phase protein. Most studies show it to have no change in concentration during an inflammatory response or its plasma concentration to decrease. A decrease in protein C could be attributed to consumption as well as a cytokines limiting the natural anticoagulant response. Activated protein C also confers a cytoprotective, anti-inflammatory, anti-apoptosis and endothelial barrier stabilisation effect when active [61].

Activated protein C signals its anti-inflammatory effects mainly via PAR-1 pathways whereby following Gi signalling and sphingosine-1-phosphate production there is improvement in endothelial cell barrier function [62].

Transcriptional profiling studies using cell cultures of human umbilical vein endothelial cells (HUVECs) have demonstrated that recombinant human activated protein C can regulate endothelial cell gene expression linked to inflammation and cell survival [63]. The activated protein C suppresses NFκB a cell nuclear transcription factor, and by reducing its expression and function this in turn causes inhibition of cytokine signaling [64].

6.2. Cytokines

Cyotkines are a superfamily of molecules involved in cell signalling many of which are increased greater than 1000-fold during an inflammatory insult. Cytokines such as interleukin (IL)-6, but also platelet-derived growth factor and monocyte chemoattractant protein (MCP)-1 are capable of stimulating tissue factor expression in mononuclear cells. Tissue factor being the initiator of thrombin generation and fibrin formation.

IL-6 is a multifunctional cytokine that is induced in many disease states such as sepsis, endotoxaemia and in-vitro after administration of tumor necrosis factor (TNF). Several studies have suggested IL-6 to be a potential mediator of endotoxin induced coagulation activation. This has been validated by treatment of chimpanzees with a monoclonal anti-IL6 antibody that ablated the activation of coagulation [65]. Cytokines are pivotal in providing a means of cross talk between inflammation and coagulation [66].

Inflammation and coagulation can not be considered as two separate processes because there are several interlocking points making them a unique defensive host reaction. The endothelium is one of the major links between the two since damaged endothelium during inflammation represents a surface where proteins involved in both coagulation and fibrinolysis and the development of inflammation are expressed. Cytokines down regulate the surface receptor thrombomodulin and the activation of protein C but at the same time increase the expression of tissue factor. Platelets adhere to these sites of vascular damage and when activated also release several cytokine mediators of inflammation, adhesion molecules and growth factors including IL-1β, CD40 ligand, vitronectin and RANTES [13], [67].

In addition to the inflammatory cytokines like interleukin 1 and TNF, infection per se can trigger the release of neutrophil extracellular traps (NETs). Which in turn release cytokines and microparticles exacerbating the acute phase haemostatic response [68].

Cytokines also upregulate the complement system activated C5b9 complexes can assemble clot promoting membrane phospholipids, TNF-α downregulates thrombomodulin and vascular heparin sulphates promoting a procoagulant environment. The net effect of this is to further lessen the inhibitory mechanisms that control thrombin generation.

6.3. Platelets

Platelet numbers increase following surgery, trauma and sepsis following a inflammatory response. Both IL-6 and thrombopoetin stimulate the production of platelets [69]. This reactive thrombocytosis can last up to13 days post surgery and may responsible for PAF adverse events in liver reperfusion and thrombotic complications post cardiac surgery. It appears that thrombopoietin is an acute phase reactant but not uniquely responsible for the rise in the platelet count during a reactive thrombocytosis but is probably aided and abetted by IL-6 [70].

Platelets release CD40 ligand which induces tissue factor expression and increases inflammatory cytokines IL-6 and IL-8. (Esmon CT). The CD40 ligand is a transmembrane protein related to TNF-α which was originally identified on stimulated $CD4^+$ T cells. The interaction of CD40 on T and B cells is integral to the development and function of the humoral immune response. It is now known that CD40 ligand is found on many cells including macrophages, endothelial cells and platelets. Upon activation platelets express CD40L within seconds. As wtih TNF-α and IL-1 the CD40L on platelets induces endothelial cells to exude cytokines and up regulate the expression of adhesion molecules. This all increases the general recruitment of leukocytes to the site of injury. Platelets therefore directly initiate the inflammatory response at the vessel wall [14]. Figure 6

The concept that platelets play a key role in the host defence and inflammatory response has taken longer to realise mainly due to their role in primary haemostasis. This new role of platelets as immune effector cells is enhanced by the finding that platelets directly interact with microbes and bacteria.

Platelet activation along with procoagulant events and fibrin formation seem crucial for the containment and killing of bacteria. Platelets have recently been shown to induce the formation of neutrophil extracellulat traps (NETs). NETs are lattice arrangements of decondensed nuclear

http://dx.doi.org/10.5772/55998

chromatin which are laced with histones that have antimicrobial properties. It also appears that this may be an 'overshooting' of the hosts defence mechanism with further platelet activation, thrombosis and endothelial cell injury [71], [72], [73].

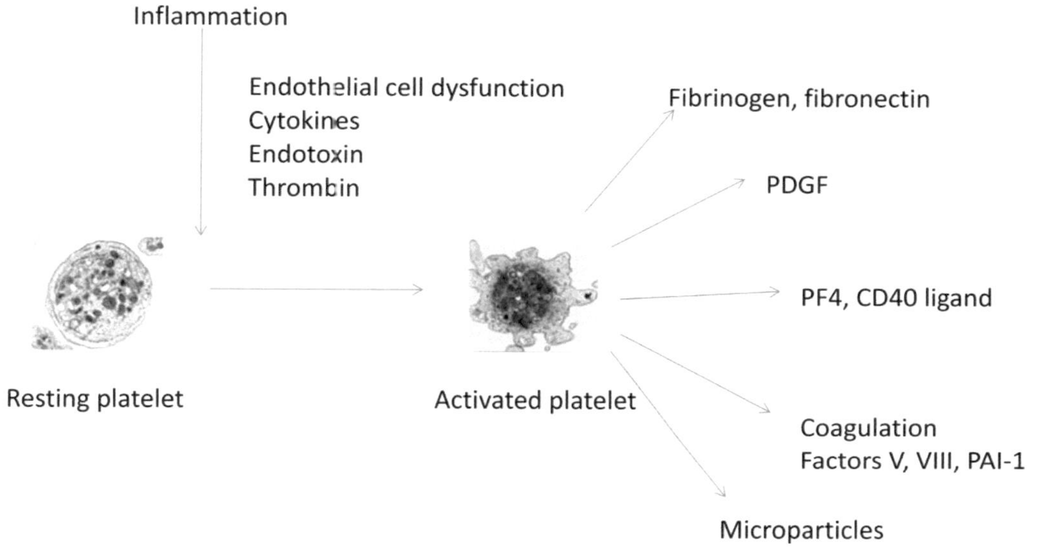

Figure 6. Inflammation and platelet activation. Platelet derived growth factor – PDGF, platetlet factor 4 – PF4.

6.4. Endothelium

Endothelial cells in the vasculature are actively involed in haemostasis providing an anticoagulant surface preventing activation of the coagulation system. Endothelial cells produce elements with proinflammatory, procoagulant and antifibrinolytic properties as well as those with the opposite anti-inflammatory, anticoagulant and profibrinolytic properties. When endothelial cells are activated or damaged they release into the local surroundings procoagulant components such as von Willebrand factor (a platelet binding factor and a carrier protein for factor VIII) and thromboxane A2 (a platelet activator) and plasminogen activator inhibitor (PAI-1 a potent inhibitor of tissue plasmingen activator). The opposite is true of components that provide an anticoagulant surface in the milieu of the blood vascular barrier. Thrombomodulin, a thrombin binding transmembrane protein that switches thrombin from a procoagulant enzyme to one that activates protein C, a nautral anticoagulant that inhibits the activity of factors V and VIII, in internalised within the endothelial cell. Thrombomodulin is also cleaved from the endothelium by activated Neutrophils. Tissue factor is expressed on the cell surface along with adhesion molecules that mediate the interaction of neutrophils and platelets these included vascular cell adhesion molecule (VCAM-1), P and E selectin and intracellular cell adhesion molecule (ICAM-1) all of which promote the inflammatory response. So the endothelium serves as an interface for the inflammatory response leading to local activation of the coagulation system, vasodilatation and pro-inflammatory state [3], [57].

6.5. Complement

Complement is part of the innate immune system and the effector of antibody mediated immunity. The biological functions of complement include the defence against infections and the clearance of immune complexes and apoptotic cells. The complement cascade is made up of approximately 30 proteins circulating in plasma and expressed on cellular surfaces. The complement cascade is activated via three pathways: classical, lectin and alternative. The classical pathway is initiated by the binding of C1q to antigen–antibody complexes. The lectin pathway is initiated via the binding of mannose-binding lectin or ficolins to sugars found at the bacterial cell wall. Both of these pathways lead to the formation of a C3 convertase. The alternative pathway is stimulated by spontaneous hydrolysis of internal thioester bonds within C3. C3a and C5a are anaphylatoxins and inflammatory mediators which are inhibited by TAFI.

Complement and coagulation are again two systems that cannot be viewed separately during an inflammatory response. Complement contributes significantly to the prothrombotic state during inflammation. The direct procoagulant activities of complement involve the activation of platelets via C3a and the C5b-9 membrane attack complex and the upregulation of tissue factor and PAI-1 expression on various cell types by C5b. Thrombin has also recently been identified as an activator of C5 linked to the coexistence of a C5 convertase enzyme [74], [75], [76].

It is of interest to note the complement factor C4B-binding protein is a positive acute phase protein that can increase greater than 400% during inflammatory states. The C4B-bp in normal circumstances binds the natural anticoagulant protein S. Protein S acts as a co-factor with activated protein C in the inactivation of factors V and VIII. It was thought that an increase in C4B-bp may increase the binding of circulating protein S, approximately 60% of protein S is normally bound leaving the other 45% free protein S to aid in the V and VIII inactivation. However this increase is restricted to the C4BPα+ form, which does not bind to PS. Therefore, the blood levels of the active free form of PS remain stable even during an acute phase response. The normal binding of protein S to C4B-bp probably allows this complex to bind via protein S high affinity for negatively charged phospholipids depositing it at area of cellular damage and limiting further apoptosis through complement activation as it will block C4b (see Protein S).

Author details

Simon J. Davidson

Department of Haematology, Royal Brompton Hospital, London, UK

References

[1] Lipinski S, Bremer L, Lammers T, Thieme F, Schreiber S, Rosenstiel P.Coagulation and inflammation. Molecular insights and diagnostic implications.Hamostaseologie. 2011;31:94-104.

[2] Levi M, van der Poll T, Büller HR.Bidirectional relation between inflammation and coagulation Circulation. 2004;109:2698-2704.

[3] Margetic S. Inflammation and haemostasis. Biochemica Medica. 2012;22:49-62.

[4] Esmon CT. Inflammtion and thrombosis. J Thromb Haemost 2003;1:1343-1348.

[5] MacFarlane RG. An enzyme cascade in the blood clotting mechanism and its function as a biochemical amplifier. Nature. 1964;202:498-499.

[6] Davie EW, Ratnoff OD. Waterfall sequence for intrinsic blood clotting. Science. 1964;145:1310-1312.

[7] Munroe DM, Hoffman M, Roberts HR. Platelets and thrombin generation. ATVB. 2002;22:1381-1389.

[8] Price GC, Thompson SA, Kam PCA. Tissue factor and tissue factor pathway inhibitor. Anaesthesia2004;59: 483–492

[9] Esmon CT, Xu J, Lupu F. Innate immunity and coagulation. J Thromb Haemost. 2011;9 (suppl.1):182-188.

[10] Levi M The coagulant response in sepsis and inflammation. Hamostaseologie. 2010;30:10-16

[11] Ma L, Dorling A. The roles of thrombin and protease-activated receptors in inflammation.Semin Immunopathol. 2012 ;34:63-72.

[12] Butenas S, Orefo T, Mann KG. Tissue factor in coagulation. Which? Where? When? Arterioscler Thromb Vasc Biol 2009;29:1989-1996.

[13] Vieira-de-Abreu A, Campbell RA, Weyrich AS, Zimmerman GA. Platelets: versatile effector cells in hemostasis, inflammation, and the immune continuum. Semin Immunopathol. 2012 ;34:5-30.

[14] Delvaeye M, Conway EM. Coagulation and innate immune responses: can we view them separately? Blood 2009;114:2367-2374

[15] Ceciliani F, Giordano A, Spagnolo V. The systemic reaction during inflammation: the acute-phase proteins.Protein Pept Lett. 2002;9:211-223

[16] Gabay C, Kushner I. Acute phase proteins and other systemic responses to inflammation. NEJM. 1999;340:448-454.

[17] Vary TC, Kimball SR. Regulation of hepatic protein synthesis in chronic inflammation and sepsis. Am J Physiol. 1992;262:445-452.

[18] Davalos D, Akassoglou K.Fibrinogen as a key regulator of inflammation in disease. Semin Immunopathol. 2012;34:43-62

[19] Medcalf RL. Fibrinolysis, inflammation and regulation of the plasminogen activating system. J Thromb Haemost. 2007;5 (suppl 1):132-142.

[20] Jennewein C, Tran N, Paulus P, Ellinghaus P, Eble JA, Zacharowski K. Novel aspects of fibrin(ogen) fragments during inflammation. Mol Med. 2011;17:568-573.

[21] van den Berg HM, De Groot PH, Fischer K. Phenotypic heterogeneity in severe hemophilia. J Thromb Haemost. 2007;5 Suppl 1:151-156.

[22] O'Donnell J, Mumford AD, Manning RA, Laffan MA. Marked elevation of thrombin generation in patients with elevated FVIII:C and venous thromboembolism. Br J Haematol. 2001;115:687-691.

[23] Rosendaal FR. High levels of factor VIII and venous thrombosis. Thromb Haemost. 2000 ;83:1-2

[24] Tichelaar V, Mulder A, Kluin-Nelemans H, Meijer K. The acute phase reaction explains only a part of initially elevated factor VIII:C levels: a prospective cohort study in patients with venous thrombosis. Thromb Res 2012;129:183-186.

[25] Rezende SM, Simmonds RE, Lane DA. Coagulation, inflammation, and apoptosis: different roles for protein S and the protein S-C4b binding protein complex. Blood. 2004;103:1192-1201.

[26] Esmon CT. Role of coagulation inhibitors in inflammation.Thromb Haemost. 2001;86:51-56

[27] Kask L, Trouw LA, Dahlbäck B, Blom AM. The C4b-binding protein-protein S complex inhibits the phagocytosis of apoptotic cells.J Biol Chem. 2004;279:23869-23873.

[28] Trouw LA, Nilsson SC, Gonçalves I, Landberg G, Blom AM. C4b-binding protein binds to necrotic cells and DNA, limiting DNA release and inhibiting complement activation. J Exp Med. 2005;201:1937-1948.

[29] Lee JA, Cochran BJ, Labov S, Ransom M. Forty Years Later and the Role of Plasminogen Activator Inhibitor Type 2/SERPINB2 Is Still an Enigma. Semin Thromb Hemost. 2011;37:395-407

[30] Cozen AE, Moriwaki H, Kremen M, DeYoung MB, Dichek HL, Slezicki KI, Young SG, Véniant M, Dichek DA. Macrophage-targeted overexpression of urokinase causes accelerated atherosclerosis, coronary artery occlusions, and premature death.Circulation. 2004;109:2129-2135.

[31] Shushakova N, Eden G, Dangers M, Menne J, Gueler F, Luft FC, Haller H, Dumler I. The urokinase/urokinase receptor system mediates the IgG immune complex-induced inflammation in lung. J Immunol. 2005 Sep 15;175(6):4060-8.

[32] Sitrin RG, Shollenberger SB, Strieter RM, Gyetko MR. Endogenously produced urokinase amplifies tumor necrosis factor-alpha secretion by THP-1 mononuclear phagocytes. J Leukoc Biol. 1996;59:302-311.

[33] Brantly M. A1-antitrypsin: not just an antiprotease. Am J Respir Cell Mol Biol. 2002;27:652-654.

[34] Borth W. Alpha 2-macroglobulin, a multifunctional binding protein with targeting characteristics. FASEB J. 1992;6:3345-3453.

[35] Zeerleder S. C1-inhibitor: more than a serine protease inhibitor. Semin Thromb Hemost. 2011;37:362-374.

[36] Davis AE 3rd, Lu F, Mejia P. C1 inhibitor, a multi-functional serine protease inhibitor. Thromb Haemost. 2010;104:886-893

[37] Bernardo A, Ball C, Nolasco L, Moake JF, Dong JF. Effects of inflammatory cytokines on the release and cleavage of the endothelial cell-derived ultralarge von Willebrand factor multimers under flow. Blood. 2004;104:100-106.

[38] Cermak J, Key NS, Bach RR, Balla J, Jacob HS, Vercellotti GM. C-reactive protein induces human peripheral blood monocytes to synthesize tissue factor.Blood. 1999;82:513-520.

[39] Boudjeltia KZ, Piagnerelli M, Brohee D, Guillaume M, Cauchie P, Vincent JL, Remacle C, Bouckaert Y, Vanhaeverbeek M. Relationship between CRP and hypofibrinolysis: Is this a possible mechanism to explain the association between CRP and outcome in critically ill patients? Thrombosis Journal. 2004;2:1-5.

[40] Filep JG. Platelets affect the structure and function of C-reactive protein. Circ Res. 2009;105:109-111.

[41] Toh CH, Samis J, Downey C, Walker J, Becker L, Brufatto N, Tejidor L, Jones G, Houdijk W, Giles A, Koschinsky M, Ticknor LO, Paton R, Wenstone R, Nesheim M. Biphasic transmittance waveform in the APTT coagulation assay is due to the formation of a Ca(++)-dependent complex of C-reactive protein with very-low-density lipoprotein and is a novel marker of impending disseminated intravascular coagulation. Blood. 2002;100:2522-2529.

[42] Niessen RW, Lamping RJ, Jansen PM, Prins MH, Peters M, Taylor FB Jr, de Vijlder JJ, ten Cate JW, Hack CE, Sturk A.Antithrombin acts as a negative acute phase protein as established with studies on HepG2 cells and in baboons. Thromb Haemost. 1999;78:1088-1092.

[43] Bourin J, Lindahl U. Glycosaminoglycans and the regulation of blood coagulation. Biochem J. 1993;289:313-330.

[44] Klein, N.J., Shennan, G.I., Heyderman, R.S. & Levin, M. Alteration in glycosaminoglycan metabolism and surface charge on human umbilical vein endothelial cells induced by cytokines, endotoxin and neutrophils. Journal of Cell Science, 1992;102, 821–832.

[45] Ostrovsky L, Woodman RC, Payne D, Teoh D, Kubes P.Antithrombin III prevents and rapidly reverses leukocyte recruitment in ischemia/reperfusion.Circulation. 1997;96:2302-2310.

[46] Mizutani A, Okajima K, Uchiba M, Isobe H, Harada N, Mizutani S, Noguchi T.Antithrombin reduces ischemia/reperfusion-induced renal injury in rats by inhibiting leukocyte activation through promotion of prostacyclin production. Blood. 2003;101:3029-3036.

[47] Altieri, D.C., Morrissey, J.H. &Edgington, T.S. (1988) Adhesive receptor Mac-1 coordinates the activation of factor X on stimulated cells of monocytic and myeloid differentiation: An alternativeinitiation of the coagulation protease cascade. Proc Natl Acad Sci U S A. 1988; 85:7462-7466

[48] Souter PJ, Thomas S, Hubbard AR, Poole S, Römisch J, Gray EAntithrombin inhibits lipopolysaccharide-induced tissue factor and interleukin-6 production by mononuclear cells, human umbilical vein endothelial cells, and whole blood. Crit Care Med. 2001;29:134-139.

[49] Poon IK, Patel KK, Davis DS, Parish CR, Hulett MD. Histidine-rich glycoprotein: the Swiss Army knife of mammalian plasma. Blood. 2011;117:2093-2101.

[50] Morrissey JH. Taking the brakes off? Blood. 2011;117:3939-3940

[51] MacQuarrie JL, Stafford AR, Yau JW, Leslie BA, Vu TT, Fredenburgh JC, Weitz JI. Histidine-rich glycoprotein binds factor XIIa with high affinity and inhibits contact-initiated coagulation. Blood 2011 ;117:4134-4141.

[52] Conway EM. Thrombomodulin and its role in inflammation.Semin Immunopathol. 2012;34:107-125.

[53] Nan B, Yang H, Yan S, Lin PH, Lumsden AB, Yao Q, Chen C. C-reactive protein decreases expression of thrombomodulin and endothelial protein C receptor in human endothelial cell. Surgery. 2005;138:212-222.

[54] Ito T, Maruyama I. Thrombomodulin: protectorate God of the vasculature in thrombosis and inflammation. J Thromb Haemost. 2011; 9 (Suppl. 1): 168–173.

[55] Mosnier LO. Platelet factor 4 inhibits thrombomodulin-dependent activation of thrombin-activatable fibrinolysis inhibitor (TAFI) by thrombin.J Biol Chem. 2011;286:502-510.

[56] Bae JS, Yang L, Rezaie AR. Receptors of the protein C activation and activated protein C signaling pathways are colocalized in lipid rafts of endothelial cells. Proc Natl Acad Sci U S A. 2007;104:2867-2872.

[57] van Hinsbergh VWM. Endothelium – role in the regulation of coagulation and inflammation. Semin Immunopathol. 2012;34:93-106.

[58] Boffa MB, Hamill JD, Maret D, Brown D, Scott ML, Nesheim ME, Koschinsky ML. Acute phase mediators modulate thrombin-activable fibrinolysis inhibitor (TAFI) gene expression in HepG2 cells. J Biol Chem. 2003;278:9250-9257.

[59] Myles T, Nishimura T, Yun TH, Nagashima M, Morser J, Patterson AJ, Pearl RG, Leung LL. Thrombin activatable fibrinolysis inhibitor, a potential regulator of vascular inflammation. J Biol Chem. 2003;278:51059-51067

[60] Skeppholm M, Wallén NH, Mobarrez F, Sollevi A, Soop A, Antovic JP. Inflammation and thrombin generation cause increased thrombin activatable fibrinolysis inhibitor levels in experimental human endotoxemia. Blood Coagul Fibrinolysis. 2009;20:611-613.

[61] Esmon CT. Protein C anticoagulant system – anti-inflammatory effects. Semin Immunopathol. 2012;34:127-132.

[62] Danese S, Vetrano S, Zhang L, Poplis VA, Castellino FJ.The protein C pathway in tissue inflammation and injury: pathogenic role and therapeutic implications Blood. 2010;115:1121-1130.

[63] Joyce DE, Gelbert L, Ciaccia A, DeHoff B, Grinnell BW. Gene expression profile of antithrombotic protein c defines new mechanisms modulating inflammation and apoptosis. J Biol Chem. 2001;276:11199-11203.

[64] Mosnier LO, Zlokovic BV, Griffin JH. The cytoprotective protein C pathway. Blood. 2007;109:3161-3172.

[65] Levi M, van Der POLL T, ten CATE H, Kuipers B, Biemond BJ, Jansen HM, ten CATE JW. Differential effects of anti-cytokine treatment on bronchoalveolar hemostasis in endotoxemic chimpanzees. Am J Respir Crit Care Med. 1998;158:92-98.

[66] de Jong HK, van der Poll T, Wiersinga WJ. The systemic pro-inflammatory response in sepsis. J Innate Immun. 2010;2:422-430.

[67] Henn V, Slupsky JR, Gräfe M, Anagnostopoulos I, Förster R, Müller-Berghaus G, Kroczek RA.CD40 ligand on activated platelets triggers an inflammatory reaction of endothelial cells. Nature. 1998;391:591-594.

[68] Borissoff JI, ten Cate H. From neutrophil extracellular traps release to thrombosis: an overshooting host-defense mechanism?J Thromb Haemost. 2011;9:1791-1794.

[69] Kaser A, Brandacher G, Steurer W, Kaser S, Offner FA, Zoller H, Theurl I, Widder W, Molnar C, Ludwiczek O, Atkins MB, Mier JW, Tilg H. Interleukin-6 stimulates

thrombopoiesis through thrombopoietin: role in inflammatory thrombocytosis. Blood. 2001;98:2720-2725.

[70] Klinger MH, Jelkmann W. Role of blood platelets in infection and inflammation. J Interferon Cytokine Res. 2002;22:913-922.

[71] Müller F, Mutch NJ, Schenk WA, Smith SA, Esterl L, Spronk HM, Schmidbauer S, Gahl WA, Morrissey JH, Renné T. Platelet polyphosphates are proinflammatory and procoagulant mediators in vivo. Cell. 2009;139:1143-1156

[72] Morrissey JH, Choi SH, Smith SA. Polyphosphate: an ancient molecule that links platelets, coagulation, and inflammation. Blood. 2012;119:5972-5979

[73] Caudrillier A, Kessenbrock K, Gilliss BM, Nguyen JX, Marques MB, Monestier M, Toy P, Werb Z, Looney MR. Platelets induce neutrophil extracellular traps in transfusion-related acute lung injury. J Clin Invest. 2012;122:2661-2671

[74] Oikonomopoulou K, Ricklin D, Ward PA, Lambris JD. Interactions between coagulation and complement--their role in inflammation.Semin Immunopathol. 2012;34:151-165.

[75] Markiewski MM, Nilsson B, Ekdahl KN, Mollnes TE, Lambris JD. Complement and coagulation: strangers or partners in crime?Trends Immunol. 2007;28:184-192.

[76] Krisinger MJ, Goebeler V, Lu Z, Meixner SC, Myles T, Pryzdial EL, Conway EM.Thrombin generates previously unidentified C5 products that support the terminal complement activation pathway. Blood. 2012;120:1717-1725.

Chapter 3

The Role of Haptoglobin and Its Genetic Polymorphism in Cancer: A Review

Maria Clara Bicho, Alda Pereira da Silva,
Rui Medeiros and Manuel Bicho

Additional information is available at the end of the chapter

http://dx.doi.org/10.5772/56695

1. Introduction

1.1. The acute phase response (APR) and haptoglobin (Hp)

Acute phase response is a stereotyped innate nonspecific reaction of the body proceeding specific immune reactions. It´s a systemic homeostatic reaction of the organism to local and or systemic disturbances caused by infections, tissue injury, trauma, immunologic disorders and neoplasias (Ron D *et al* 1990, Trautwein C *et al* 1994, Gruys E *et al* 2005). Proinflammatory cytokines are released at the place of tissue injury, diffuses locally and systemically to the vascular system and activates receptors on different target cells resulting in the activation of hypothalamic-pituitary-adrenal axis (HPAA), results in the production of growth hormone secretion and induces changes in the concentration of several plasma proteins (Ron D *et al* 1990, Trautwein C *et al* 1994, Gruys E *et al* 2005).

These acute phase proteins (APPs) can be positive (higher levels in plasma) or negative (lower levels in plasma). The alteration on mRNA in hepatocytes is due to simultaneous influence of systemic cytokines (IL1, IL6 and TNFα), glucocorticoids and catecholamines (Bowman BH 1993, Ron D *et al* 1990, Trautwein C *et al* 1994).

Haptoglobin together with fibrinogen, α-globulins with antiprotease-activity and lipopolysaccharide binding protein belong to the group of positive APPs that increase 3-fold in mammals (Trautwein C *et al* 1994, Gruys E *et al* 2005).

Haptoglobin (Hp) is an acute phase $\alpha 2$ plasma glycoprotein that is a component of innate immunity, which also may influence acquired immunity. Through both types of immunity,

Hp is involved in the pathogenesis of tumours and infections (Langlois MR and Delanghe JR 1996, Van Vlierberghe H. *et al* 2004, Levy AP *et al* 2010).

2. Haptoglobin (Hp) synthesis, gene structure, variants and its geographic distribution

Haptoglobin locus is on chromosome 16q22 and its gene is transcribed and translated into a single peptide which undergoes post-translational processing resulting in a smaller α-chain and a longer β-chain linked by disulphide bridge (Giblett ER 1968, Langlois MR and Delanghe JR 1996, Wicher KB and Fries E 2007).

In 1955, Smithies, using thin layer starch gel electrophoresis identified the three phenotypes of Hp (1-1, 2-1, 2-2), corresponding to the α-chain length interindividual genetic variation.

The three genotypes are shown in electrophoresis in polyacrylamide gel electrophoresis (PAGE) (fig 1).

This genetic variation results from an internal duplication of a gene segment (exons 3 and 4), correspondent to α-chain of Hp1 giving rise to a larger one, characteristic of Hp2 (Maeda *et al* 1984, Wicher KB and Fries E 2007).

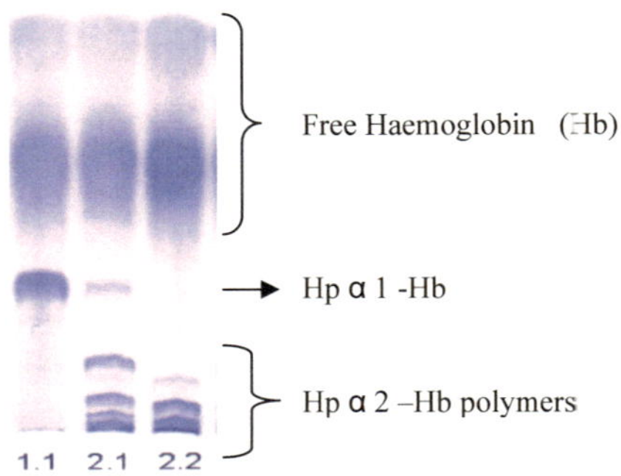

Figure 1. Typical pattern of haptoglobin bands in a polyacrylamide gel electrophoresis (PAGE). Shown are the phenotypes: Hp 1-1, is characterized by a fast migration band; Hp 2-2 is characterized by slower multiple bands; Hp 2-1, characterized by a mixed pattern of two allelic forms. The ultrafast bands are no haptoglobin bound haemoglobin chains (Linke RP 1984, Guerra J *et al* 1997).

This inter-individual variation is found only in humans and aroused about 100,000 years ago in Southeast Asia. The great majority of other mammals have only one band corresponding to the human Hp1-1, except the sheep, deer and cows (Ruminantia), which have only slow bands corresponding to Hp2-2 (Bowman BH and Kurosky A 1982, Wicher KB and Fries 2007).

The appearance of Hp2 can represent an important evolutionary genetic contribution for interpopulational diversity in human pathology (ER Giblett 1968, Maeda et al 1984, Wicher KB and Fries 2007). This allele is predominant in the human population (about 80% in some ethnic groups) and Hp1 allele is more predominant in populations subjected to malaria burden (Giblett ER 1968, Langlois MR and Delanghe JR 1996, Wobeto VP et al 2008, Levy AP et al 2010).

In close linkage with haptoglobin gene there is another one, 2-2 Kb downstream from Hp locus, coding for Hp related (Hpr) plasma protein with 91% sequence identity to Hp1. The α-chain of Hpr contains a hydrophobic signal peptide that may explain its association to lipoprotein particles (HDL) or membranes (Kuhajda FP *et al* 1989 a, b).

3. Haptoglobin locals of its synthesis and regulation

The Hp gene is expressed primarily in hepatocytes and more recently has been described in other locations, such as keratinocytes, airway epithelial cells of lung, leucocytes, fibrocytes, adipocytes and endometrial cells, particularly during the blastocyst implantation (Friederichs WE *et al* 1995, Olson EG *et al* 1997 Wang *et al* 2005, Shaw JL *et al* 2007, Yang F 2000 *et al*, Larsen K *et al* 2006, and Theilgaard-Mönch K *et al* 2006).

Haptoglobin synthesis is induced by cytokines such as interleukin-6 (IL-6), interleukin-1 (IL-1) and tumour necrosis factor (TNFα) released by the macrophages, after activation of the innate immunity cells by PAMPs (pathogen associated molecular patterns) such as lipopolysaccharide, a TLR4 (Toll Like Receptor) activator (Raynes JG et al 1991, Kaisho T and Alkira S 2002).

Glucocorticoids and catecholamines activate haptoglobin synthesis previously induced by interleukins (increased), whereas insulin exerts an opposite action, despite the presence of these interleukins (Ron D et al 1990, Campos SP and Baumann H 1992 Nascimento CO et al 2004, Gruys E et al 2005 and XiaLi-xin et al 2008). Hypoxia also induces indirectly its synthesis (Wenger RH et al 1995, Oh Mi-Kyung et al 2011).

4. Haptoglobin metabolism, actions and respective mechanisms

Haptoglobin has a pronounced anti-inflammatory action, which is explained by its ability to bind to heme of haemoglobin, forming a Hp-Hb complex. This is characterized by stability and high affinity to its specific type scavenger receptor (CD163) located in the hepatocyte and the phagocytic-type cells such as circulating monocytes, resident macrophages (M2) and liver Kupffer cells. The CD163 is a membrane protein 130-kDa, whose long extracellular region has nine cysteine-rich domains of scavenger-type receptor (Graversen JH *et al* 2002, Nielsen MJ *et al* 2010, Akila P *et al* 2012). The expression of receptors (CD 163), Hp and hemoxygenase (HO-1), is strongly activated by antinflammatory cytokines, such as interleukins (IL6, IL10), growth factors (M-CSF) and glucocorticoids (Moestrup SK and Møller H 2004). In contrast CD 163 is down regulated by IL4 and GM-CSF, Interferon γ and TNF (Nielsen MJ *et al* 2010, Vallelian F *et al* 2011 and Akila P *et al* 2012).

After binding to its receptor the Hp-Hb complex is internalized in the form of endosome, followed by fusion with lysosomes, proteolysis of globin and intracellular release of heme to hemoxygenase (HO-1) with concomitant formation of biliverdin that is converted in bilirrubin, CO (carbon monoxide) and release of iron to ferritin where is compartmentalised (Graversen JH *et al* 2002, Nielsen MJ *et al* 2010, Vallelian F *et al* 2011, Akila P *et al* 2012).

The small protein Hp1-1 is excreted in the urine when occurs kidney damage, however, the Hp2-1 and Hp2-2 are always retained (Fagoonee S 2005). The clearance of free haemoglobin (Hb) after intravascular haemolysis by the haptoglobin is higher in individuals carrying the Hp1 allele (Giblett ER 1968, Langlois MR and Delanghe JR 1996, Moestrup SK and Møller H 2004, Nielsen MJ *et al* 2010, Vallelian F *et al* 2011, Akila P *et al* 2012).

The free Hb has the ability to catalyse the formation of hydroxyl radicals (OH·), from the hydrogen peroxide, with highly damaging effects to the cellular constituents and extracellular macromolecules (Sadrzadeh SMH 1984, Gutteridge JMC 1987).

The Hp-Hb complex, reduces the loss of Hb in urine and concomitant loss of iron and its transport is done mainly to the liver. As a result, the removal of free Hb has much important consequences for the organisms, preventing renal injury that may occur when the free Hb passes through the glomerular filter (Fagoonee S *et al* 2005). Also Hp prevents the promotion of free radicals and its accumulation in endothelial cells, catalysed by heme, where it causes vessel injury (Nielsen MJ *et al* 2010, Vallelian F *et al* 2011 and Akila P *et al* 2012). However, there is a great variability in these responses, which is dependent of Hp polymorphism having individuals with the Hp2-2 a lower antioxidant capacity than those with other phenotypes. Furthermore at the extra-vascular interstitial level, the antioxidant capacity of carriers of Hp2-2 is lower, because of its higher molecular mass that restricts its extravascular diffusion (Langlois MR and Delanghe JR 1996, Van Vierberghe *et al* 2004, Fagoonee S. *et al* 2005, Levy AP *et al* 2010).

Levels of haptoglobin in plasma or serum are lower in healthy infants than adults whose concentrations are between 0.38 and 2.08g/l (Langlois MR and Delanghe JR 1996). These steady state levels are consequence of haptoglobin half-life of 3.5 days and Hp-Hb complex of ten minutes (Sadrzadeh SMH and Bozorgmehr J 2004). The Hp can also be detected in urine and other organic fluids (Langlois MR and Delanghe JR 1996, Sadrzadeh SMH and Bozorgmehr J 2004). The half-life of Hp-Hb complex is phenotype dependent being Hp1-1 shorter than Hp2-2 (Levy AP *et al* 2010). Plasma concentrations are also phenotype dependent, people with Hp1-1 having the highest, Hp2-1 intermediate and Hp2-2 lesser concentrations in plasma (Langlois MR and Delanghe JR 1996).

Haptoglobin levels are quantified by chemical and immunochemical methods, from these the most utilised are the immunonephelometric and immunoturbidimetric methods that are automated (Langlois MR and Delanghe JR 1996, Sadrzadeh SMH and Bozorgmehr J 2004).

The haptoglobin polymorphism is most commonly determined by starch or polyacrylamide electrophoresis (Fig 1). When plasma levels are lower than 0.10g/l PCR based assays are utilised (Linke RP 1984, Langlois MR and Delanghe JR 1996, Guerra A *et at* 1997, Levy AP *et al* 2010). More recently in both, levels measurement and phenotype, are utilised new proteomic methods based on two dimensional gel electrophoresis and quantitative determination by mass spectrometry (MALDI-TOF-MS and SELDI-TOF-MS) methods (Gast M-C *et al* 2008, Chen C-B *et al* 2008).

The Hp-Hb complex also binds nitric oxide or nitrogen monoxide (NO), produced by cytokine activated macrophages, thus preventing their physiological and pathological actions (Langlois MR and Delanghe JR 1996, Azarov I *et al* 2008, Alayash A 2011). Also this action is phenotype dependent, because Hp2-2/Hb complex scavenge more NO than Hp1-1/Hb due to its longer half-life (Azarov I *et al* 2008, Levy AP *et al* 2010, Alayash A 2011).

The Hp is also a potent endogenous inhibitor of prostaglandin synthesis, resulting in anti-inflammatory action. The inhibitory effects of Hp2-2 and Hp2-1 are less pronounced than those of Hp1-1 (Kendall PA *et al* 1979, Langlois MR and Delanghe JR 1996, Saeed SA *et al* 2007).

Haptoglobin has also bacteriostatic effects, because the capture and compartmentalization of the iron of Hb made it no longer available for bacterial growth. The Hp 2-2 is more efficient than the other phenotypes in this action against *Streptococcus*. There are also microorganisms that can remove iron from the Hp-Hb complex (Langlois MR and Delanghe JR 1996, Weinberg ED 1996, Van Vlierberghe *et al* 2004).

The role of Hp in angiogenesis has been identified as one of the factors for modulation of differentiation and proliferation of endothelial cells during the formation of new vessels (Cid MC *et al* 1993, Park SJ 2009). Free Hb can promote indirectly carcinogenesis through the iron that is necessary for cell growth. The withholding of iron inhibits cell growth and depresses the immune system (Langlois MR and Delanghe JR 1996, Weinberg ED 1996).

The local increased concentration of Hp in chronic inflammatory processes is important for the ischemic tissue reparation, promoting collateral vessel formation. Of the three genetic forms Hp2.2 is the most angiogenic (Cid MC *et al* 1993).

In resident tissues macrophages (M2 type), carbon monoxide (CO) resulting from the intracellular degradation Hp-Hb complex appears to be involved in anti-inflammatory effects of interleukin 10 (IL-10). The suppression of these immune and inflammatory responses results from its ability to decrease the antigen presentation and cytokine synthesis. This mechanism of regulation is more active in patients with the Hp1-1 phenotype that has a greater clearance of their complexes with their CD163 receptors present on monocytes, than for those carrying the phenotype Hp2-2 (Nielsen MJ *et al* 2010, Vallelian F *et al* 2011 and Akila P *et al* 2012).

In macrophages, after the endocytosis of the Hp-Hb complex and CD163, increased levels of cytoplasmic iron ocurr, inducing the synthesis of ferritin, a primary iron storage, which can subtract it from inflammation site (Cozzi *et al* 2004). The activation of the CD 163 also induces a signal mediated by protein tyrosine kinase, leading to the secretion of anti-inflammatory cytokines and giving rise to a connection between the clearance function of the Hp and their immunomodulatory functions (Van Vlierberghe *et al* 2004, Guetta *et al* 2007, Nielsen MJ *et al* 2010, Vallelian F *et al* 2011 and Akila P *et al* 2012).

Haptoglobin can also modulate the immune response by binding to receptors on immune cells, such as CD22 on B lymphocytes and β2 integrin (CD11b/CD18) in neutrophils or LFA-1 (lymphocyte function associated antigen-1) in T lymphocytes (EL Ghmati SM *et al* 1996, Giannoni E *et al* 2003, Bottini N *et al* 2005). The Hp may bind to neutrophils, inhibiting NADPH oxidase activation and the production of reactive forms of oxygen associated with inflammation (Moestrup SK and Møller H, 2004, Guetta *et al* 2007).

Changes of the ratio of lymphocytes Th1 and Th2 are important for the determination of susceptibility to viral and parasitic infections, for allergies, for antitumor responses and autoimmunity (Gleeson ME 2006, Clerici M *et al* 1998). It was shown that Hp plays a modulating role of the Th1/Th2 ratio, promoting a Th2 dominant response, which is more pronounced in patients with the Hp1-1 and 2-1 phenotypes (Bottini N *et al* 2005, Guetta *et al* 2007).

The objective of this chapter is to review the scientific evidence of haptoglobin role, as an immune innate protein in the several aspects of cancer biology and its possible clinical importance as a genetic and a circulating biomarker for that pathology.

The methodology for this review is based in the search in the literature of relevant studies in cancer concerning both the circulating levels of haptoglobin (including the recent described fucosylated glicans), haptoglobin related (Hpr) and the genetic variation studies, in the Medline Data Bases and the related papers, since the first reports in the sixties of the last century until actuality. A special attention will be a consideration of cancer associated with human papillomavirus (HPV). The keywords used in the search will be haptoglobin, cancer genetics, circulating levels and clinics.

5. Haptoglobin (Hp) and its related pathway as biomarkers in cancer

Genetic polymorphism of haptoglobin leads to its functional differences resulting in interindividual variation of the related intermediate phenotypes at the different biological levels that can constitute circulating biological markers of clinical importance not only for the susceptibility but also for the prognostic and response to treatment at the diverse levels of natural history of the neoplasia disease (Bicho MC 2011). We will review by organs and systems the studies that evidence those aspects.

In table 1, we describe the association of Hp polymorphism in several populations with CNS head and neck, lung, blood and skin malignancies.

For the central nervous system it was demonstrated that haptoglobin is transcribed and expressed (proteomic methods) in human glioblastome cells and it is significantly associated with greater plasmatic levels in the higher grades compared with lower ones and those of control subjects (Sanchez DJ *et al* 2001, Kumar DM *et al* 2010). Also it was demonstrated that Hp increases in vitro glioblastome cell migration (Kumar DM *et al* 2010), table 1.

Head and neck squamous cell cancer (HNSCC) is a term that collectively refers to cancer of oral cavity, salivary glands, larynx and pharynx. After a first study the authors whose objective is discovery of circulating biomarkers associated with those tumours, demonstrate in HNSCC in general and nasopharynx in particular, the haptoglobin overexpression, in a stage and tumour volume dependency (Chen C-B *et al* 2008, Lee CC *et al* 2009). Another group confirmed the involvement of the Hp phenotype in infection with Epstein-Barr virus (EBV) that is associated with nasopharynx carcinoma (Speeckaert R *et al* 2009).

In the eighties several studies of association with cancer of acute phase proteins in particular haptoglobin were done, that is the case for the lung cancer in 309 Swedish patients where the

http://dx.doi.org/10.5772/56695

Neoplasia	Population (N) (Control/Neo)	Conclusions	References
Human glioblastome	N=26/96 India	Hp2 allele higher grades	Sanchez DJ *et al* 2001; Kumar DM *et al* 2010
Head/neck squamous cell cancer	N=135/163	Hp2 allele tumour volume dependency	Chen C-B *et al* 2008
	N=134/49 Taiwan		Lee CC *et al* 2009
Nasopharynx carcinoma	N=918/208 Belgium	Hp1-1 and Hp 2-1 less prone to positive EBV serology	Speeckaert R *et al* 2009
Lung cancer	N=309 Sweden	Hp1 allele more frequent in adenocarcinoma in females	Beckman G *et al* 1986
Acute lymphoid leukemia	N=2331/110 Sweden	No association	Fröhlander N and Stendahl U 1988
Leukemias	N= 211 Israel	Associated Hp1-1 with ALL, AML, CML	Nevo S and Tatarsky I 1986
Acute myeloid leukemia	N=197/188 Brazil		Campregher PV *et al* 2004
ALL, AML, CML, IgA ML	N=134 Australia	Higher Hp 1-1 association	Mitchell RJ *et al* 1988 Germinis A et al 1983
Squamous cell carcinoma (SCC)	N=300 Belgium	Hp phenotype 1.1 more prone to develop SCC in kidney transplanted patients	Speeckaert R *et al* 2012
Kaposi´s sarcoma		Hp1.1 phenotype more prone	Speeckaert R *et al* 2011

Abbreviations: ALL-Acute lymphatic leukaemia; AML- Acute myeloid leukaemia; CML- Chronic myeloid leukaemia; CLL-Chronic lymphatic leukaemia; ML- Myeloma.

Table 1. Haptoglobin and Cancer: Various Tumours.

Hp1 allele is more frequent in women with adenocarcinoma (Beckman G *et al* 1986). More recently other group confirmed the association of local higher levels of the Hp l expression in pulmonary adenocarcinomas in opposition to squamous cell carcinomas (SCC) and small cell carcinomas (Abdullah M 2009).

There are five references for blood malignancies such as acute and chronic lymphoid leukemia and acute myeloid leukemia from three different ethnic groups Sweden, Israel and Brazil (Caucasians and Afro-descendants) and only one sample of Ashkenazy Jews (Germinis A *et al* 1983, Nevo S and Tatarsky I 1986, Mitchell RJ *et al* 1988, Fröhlander N and Stendahl U 1988, Campregher PV *et al* 2004).

Cutaneous malignancies and in particular squamous cell carcinoma (SCC)/Bowen´s disease are more frequent in kidney transplanted patients, that are more prone to disease when are carriers of Hp 1.1 phenotypes particularly after ten years of the transplantation (Speeckaert R *et al* 2012). The same happens in the development of Kaposi's sarcoma in HIV positive patients, even after adjustment for age, gender and AIDS status (Speeckaert R *et al* 2011).

Tumours of gastrointestinal tract where also studied and the single reference to haptoglobin polymorphism in colon cancer refers to one association in 184 Greek patients of Hp1-1 phenotype (Archimandritis A *et al* 1993), table 2.

More recently it was shown that Hp is produced in a large molecular complex with the beta chain of urokinase in cancer cells as well as in capillary endothelial cells (Harvey S *et al* 2009). This cancer-associated glycoform of Hp (β-chain) is a ligand for Galectin-3, a beta-galactoside binding protein implicated in tumour progression and metastases of colorectal cancers (Bresalier RS *et al* 2004).

Neoplasia	Population (N) (Control/Neo)	Conclusions	References
Colon cancer	N=2026/184 Greece	Association of Hp1-1 phenotype	Archimandritis A *et al* 1993
Gastric cancer	N=104/100 India	Risk for Hp2-2 carriers	Jayanthi M *et al* 1989
	N=114/2026 Greece	No association	Theodoropoulos G *et al* 1992
Oesophageal cancer		Higher risk for Hp2-1 phenotype	Jayanthi M *et al* 1989
Pancreatic cancer	N=11/11 China	Frequency of Hp 2-2 is higher	Deng R *et al* 2007

Table 2. Haptoglobin and Cancer: Digestive Tumours.

Geographic differences have been reported regarding the influence of the Hp alleles in cancer risk. In India, where the frequency of Hp2 allele is high at the population level (84%) the risk for gastric cancer of the Hp2-2 phenotype carriers is 4.04 and the risk for oesophageal is 3.86 for Hp2-1 phenotype carriers (Jayanthi M *et al* 1989). On the contrary in another geographic localization (Greece) a study of a similar number of gastric carcinoma patients didn't show any difference for the same polymorphism (Theodoropoulos G *et al* 1992).

Deng R *et al* demonstrated in 2007 that, in pancreatic carcinoma patients, the frequency of Hp 2-2 is higher compared with chronic pancreatitis patients and normal controls. Haptoglobin of these patients is not elevated in serum, but it is abnormally fucosylated in β-chain that has four N-glycans sites, the same happens but not so extensively in hepatocellular, gastric and colorectal carcinomas. The fucosylation of Hp seems to be induced by a factor secreted by these tumours itself (Nakano et al 2009, Miyoshi E, Nakano M 2008)

Early references of the distribution of haptoglobin polymorphism in Greek patients with prostate carcinoma compared with prostate benign hypertrophy (BPH) patients failed to

http://dx.doi.org/10.5772/56695

demonstrate any association (Germenis A *et al* 1983, Dimopoulos MA *et al* 1984). These results were consistent with a recent report from an association study realized in an African population where the Authors didn´t also demonstrate any association of the Hp polymorphism with PSA (Prostate Specific Antigen) and prostate cancer patients survival (Mavondo GA *et al* 2012). However there were demonstrated higher circulation levels of monoclonal antibodies against glycosyl epitopes presents in the beta chain of Hp in prostate carcinoma compared with BPH that decreased after radical prostatectomy (Saito S *et al* 2008), table 3.

Serum levels of haptoglobin were elevated in kidney and bladder cancer concomitantly with a metabolite of Prostaglandin F2α, however only in bladder cancer was demonstrated in 264 Germans a statistically significant lower frequency of Hp2-2 genotype (Dunzendorfer U *et al* 1981; Bemkman HG *et al* 1987).

Neoplasia	Population (N) (Control/Neo)	Conclusions	References
Prostate cancer	N=155/1´5 Greek patients	Failed to demonstrate any Hp association	Germenis A *et al* 1983; Dimopoulos MA *et al* 1984
	N=122/74 Africa, Botswana Zimbabwe	Any association of the polymorphism with PSA and survival	Mavondo GA *et al* 2012
Bladder cancer	N=264 Germany	Lower frequency of Hp 2-2	Benkman HG *et al* 1987

Table 3. Haptoglobin and Cancer: Urological Tumours.

For breast cancer despite consistency of overrepresentation of Hp 1 allele in three earlier studies (Tsamantains C *et al* 1980, Kaur H *et al* 1984, Bartel U *et al* 1985) and only one negative study (Hudson BL *et al* 1982) a more recent study demonstrate that Hp phenotype distribution in patients is family history-dependent. For these authors the frequency of Hp 1-1 and Hp 2-1 phenotypes is higher in the familial group and the opposite for the no familial group (Awadallah S and Atoum MF 2004). Moreover, in the recent study whose objective was to search for circulating proteins, predictive of recurrences and free survival of high risk primary breast cancer, with proteomic techniques (SELDI-TOF-MS) the authors, based on disturbances of iron (low levels of ferritin light chain is associated with good prognosis), identified Hp 2 allele as risk factor, nonetheless validated in an independent, sample and technique group of patients (Gast M-C W *et al* 2008). Also, it may have clinical important value, as a biomarker for recurrence in early breast cancer patients, the haptoglobin related (Hpr) protein in tissues and plasma (Kuhajda FP *et al* 1989 a-b).

The first references from the sixties of the last century about gynaecologic tumours indicate contradictory results between the authors when they were analyzed as a whole in what concerns to the frequency of Hp1 allele (Larkin MF 1967, Milunicova A *et al* 1969). However, a posterior reference of Bartel U et al 1985 confirms a higher Hp1-1 genotype frequency in 246

German patients with gynaecological and breast tumours. When only ovarian cancer samples were considered, two references, one Polish and another Swedish, indicate they are associated respectively with Hp 1 allele and Hp2-1 phenotype in patients with family history (Dobryszycka W and Wavas M. 1983, Fröhlander N and Stendahl U 1988).

Cervical neoplasia is a good model that illustrates haptoglobin and its polymorphism influence in the several steps of its natural history interacting with oncogenic and non-oncogenic HPV (Human Papillomavirus) and other co-factors such as sexual steroid hormones and smoking habits (Bicho MC 2011).

Preliminary reports on the role of this haptoglobin polymorphism in the development of cervical cancer were conflicting, with two authors (Milunicova and Bartel) indicating that Hp1 allele carriers were at risk of cancer development. In opposition, Larkin et al report the Hp2 allele as the most represented in their cervical cancer cases (Milunicova A *et al* 1969, Bartel U *et al* 1985 U, Larkin M 1967). Those reports were published previous to the, nowadays confirmed, association of oncogenic HPV types as the primary etiologic factor of cervical cancer and the HPV effect was not evaluated in the control populations. However, HPV is a necessary but not a sufficient cause of cervical cancer and it is also important the presence the other co-factors host related. One of these co-factors can be the immune response of the host. It has been proposed a role for haptoglobin a one of such co-factors (Mahmud SM *et al* 2007, Bicho MC *et al* 2006 and 2009).

In the case control study conducted in Canada (307 cases vs 358 control women), Mahmud et al examined the association of Hp phenotype with high grade cervical intraepithelial neoplasia (CIN III), a precursor lesion of invasive carcinoma (ICC). The control group had to present a normal cytology and HPV genotyping was performed to evaluate the HPV oncogenic type status. Accordingly, only when the risk analysis is restricted to the HPV positive women, an association was observed and Hp 1-1 carriers have almost a threefold increased susceptibility to the development of CIN III (OR=2.7, 95% IC: 1.0-7.2) (Mahmud SM et al 2007). In a recent study, we report an increased susceptibility for women that are Hp 1-1 carriers to develop ICC (OR=4.62, 95% IC: 1.86-11.48) (Bicho MC 2011). These results are consistent with another study performed in a different geographic localization (Ghana) and indicating a significant protective effect for the Hp2 allele in homozygous women (Quaye IK et al 2009). In another report, we studied the influence of Hp polymorphism on the risk for the development of HSIL and ICC (n=196) under the influence of sex steroid hormones. We found that the risk for an interaction is proportionally higher with the number of Hp 1 allele presents (Bicho MC et al 2009). However, when the interaction between Hp polymorphism with smoking habits was studied the Hp 2 allele in homozygoty increased the risk to develop HSIL and ICC (Bicho MC et al 2006).

6. Discussion

During the first thirty years (from the sixties to nineties of the last century) of cancer association studies, genetic blood markers, including haptoglobin were concomitantly studied with

Neoplasia	Population (N) (Control/Neo)	Conclusions	References
Breast cancer	N=109 Greece	Overrepresentation of Hp 1 allele	Tsamantains C *et al* 1980
	N=50/50 India	Overrepresentation of Hp 1 allele	Kaur H *et al* 1984
	N=246 Germany	Overrepresentation of Hp 1 allele	Bartel U *et al* 1985
	N=129/200 Jordania	Higher frequency of Hp 1 allele	Awadallah S
	Familial (N=42) Non familial (N=86)	Higher frequency of Hp 1 and Hp 2 alleles	Atoum MF 2004
	USA	No association	Hudson BL *et al* 1982
	N=371 USA	No association	Gast M-C W *et al* 2008
Ovarian cancer	N=114/132 Polland	Associated Hp 1 allele	Dobryszycka W and Wavas M. 1983
	N=182 Swedish	Associated Hp2-1 phenotype with family history	Fröhlander N and Stendahl U 1988
Cervical cancer	N=170/85 Checoslovakia	Hp1 allele carriers at risk	Milunicova A *et al* 1969
	N=430/526 Germany	Hp1 allele carriers at risk	Bartel U *et al* 1985
	N=430/526 USA	Hp2 allele as the most represented	Larkin M 1967
	N=358/307 Canada	In HPV positive women, risk for Hp 1-1 is higher CIN III	Mahmud SM *et al* 2007
	N= 396/196 Portugal	In ICC women the risk for Hp 1-1 carriers is greater in steroid hormone ingestion	Bicho MC 2011
	N=120/60 Ghana	Protective effect of the Hp2 allele in homozygoty	Quaye IK *et al* 2009

Table 4. Haptoglobin and Cancer: Gynaecological Tumours.

descriptive studies of allele distribution in the different populations (Giblett ER 1968, Langlois MR and Delanghe JR 1996, Wobeto VP *et al* 2008, Levy AP *et al* 2010). These preliminary reports usually were cross-sectional case control studies, that didn't enter in consideration with the biological plausibility in cancer linked to the genetic variation. Diverse geographic regions, with very different distribution of alleles, various genetic variations backgrounds and above all have different environments that interacts with genomes to give highly variable phenotypes, may explain controversial results.

Moreover, the lack of reproducibility of the several studies may also reflect methodological differences in the criteria of case definitions and selection of controls, and in what concerns to the influence of environment of factors such as microbiological (HPV, EBV, M. tuberculosis, H. Pylori, Plasmodia), smoking habits, sun exposition, xenobiotic and sex steroid hormones (Beckman G *et al* 1986, Benkmann HG *et al* 1987, Bicho MC *et al* 2006 and 2009, Mahmud *et al* and 2007, Abdullah M *et al* 2009, Speeckaert R *et al* 2011 and 2012).

The usual cross-sectional approach of these studies didn´t take into account the somewhat different influences of the genotypes on the natural story of the cancer that courses in multistep way (Zur Hausen H 2002). The great majority of the studies were done in patients with distant phenotypes (advanced stage cancer) and take not in consideration the subclinical disease. This isn´t evidenced in those times by lack of knowledge of physiopathology and lack of reliable biomarkers (circulating and imaging) that gives a more dynamic picture of the situation.

It was not common, the realization of measurements of serum and plasma levels of the Hp independently of phenotype in part due too time consuming of the technics (Langlois MR and Delanghe JR 1996). In these cases, not even the local processes are reflected in circulation but also it is demonstrated the existence of a local tissue environment in what Hp functions in paracrine and autocrine way (Yang F *et al* 2000, Xie Y, *et al* 2000, Sharpe-Timms *et al* 2002, Wang H *et al* 2005, Shaw JLV *et al* 2007).

The natural history of cervical cancer seems to be dependent of genetic polymorphism of haptoglobin in its interaction with HPV and cofactors such as sex steroid hormones and smoking habits (Bicho MC *et al* 2006 and 2009, Mahmud *et al* and 2007).

Also there are reports of the different influences of Hp alleles in a context of familiar history for the breast and ovarian cancers (Fröhlander N and Stendahl U 1988, Awadallah S and Atoum MF 2004).

For the clarification of these issues a better knowledge of the physiopathology mechanisms of action of the Hp alleles is necessary.

Haptoglobin as a pleiotropic protein has several different functions being the Hp1 allele and correspondent genotypes Hp1-1 and Hp1-2, the more represented in the several cancers reviewed. The innate immune response of the host against the tumour is limited in the subject's carriers of the Hp1 allele through several mechanisms, already reviewed.

It is accepted, in this pathway, the role of Hp-Hb, CD163, HO-1, CO, bilirubin, activation of anti-oxidant intracellular systems (including ferritin), and extrusion of iron through ferroportin. This pathway is characteristic of immunosuppressive tumor macrophages M2 types that are more active in Hp1 carriers inducing a switch for a Th2 antinflammatory cytokine profile characteristic of lesser Th1 type cytotoxic immune antitumor mechanisms (Van Vlierberghe *et al* 2004, Guetta *et al* 2007, Nielsen MJ *et al* 2010, Vallelian F *et al* 2011 and Akila P *et al* 2012).

This switch can be also dependent of a stronger acute phase response characteristic of Hp1 carriers that can modulate immune cells activity after binding of Hp to its receptors CD22, β2 integrin and LFA located respectively in B cells neutrophils and T cells (EL Ghmati SM *et al* 1996, Giannoni E *et al* 2003, Bottini N *et al* 1999 and 2005, Arredouani MS *et al* 2005, Lu JY *et al* 2007). A third mechanism can be the interaction of environmental factors such as sex steroid hormones and glucocorticoids that activates predominantly Th2 arm of acquired immunity in synergy with Hp1 allele as happens in cervical cancer (Gleeson M 2006, Bicho MC *et al* 2009, Akila P *et al* 2012).

An increased prevalence of Hp 2-2 genotype is observed in some tumours leading to the hypothesizes of haptoglobin involvement in the mechanisms associated with the carcinogenesis and tumorigenesis of the chronic inflammation (head and neck carcinomas, glioblastome, gastric carcinoma).

The lower antioxidative capacity and inhibition of prostaglandin synthase associated to the genotype Hp 2-2 are the best known explanatory mechanisms (Wen WN et al 2001, Saeed SA *et al* 2007). Indirect effects of prostaglandins on carcinogenesis are mediated through the stabilization of HIF1α and the resultant expression of angiogenic factors like EPO (erythropoietin), VEGF (vascular endothelial growth factor), that have synergic effects with Hp2-2 (Cid MC *et al* 1993, Liu XH *et al* 2002, Acs G *et al* 2003, Ye YN *et al* 2004, Mihailović M *et al* 2005, Palayoor ST *et al* 2009, Park SJ 2009).

Another mechanism involved is the withholding of iron in macrophages that is necessary for the proliferation of immune cell (Touitou Y *et al* 1985, Weinberg ED 1996, Cozzi A *et al* 2004).

The effects of smoking habits are modulated by Hp2-2, because the effects in the nicotine down regulation of haptoglobin expression and also the effects of CO producing local hypoxia and the immune depression (Ye YN *et al* 2005).

7. Perspectives

More studies are necessary to complete our understanding about the role of this important acute phase protein, its levels variations, particularly the fucosylated isoforms and its regulation, the Hpr and its polymorphism and its immunomodulation role in cancer. Finally, future studies may focus in the importance of haptoglobin polymorphism conducting to a pharmacogenetic approach to chemoprevention.

Author details

Maria Clara Bicho[1,2], Alda Pereira da Silva[1], Rui Medeiros[3] and Manuel Bicho[1,2]

1 Genetics Laboratory Faculty of Medicine, University of Lisbon, Portugal

2 Rocha Cabral Institute Lisbon, Portugal

3 Portuguese Institute of Oncology (IPOFG) Oporto, Portugal

References

[1] Abdullah M, Schultz H, Kähler D, Branscheid D, Dalhoff K, Zabel P, Vollmer E, Goldmann. Expression of the acute phase protein haptoglobin in human lung cancer and tumor-free lung tissues. Pathology Research and Pratice. 2009: 623-647

[2] Acs G, Zhang PJ, Mcgrath CM, Asc P, Mcbroom J, Mohyeldin A, Liu S, Lu H, Verma A. Hypoxia-inducible erythropoietin signalling in squamous dysplasia and squamous cell carcinoma of uterine cervix and its potential role in cervical carcinogenesis and tumor progression. Am J Pathol 2003; 162(69): 1789-1806

[3] Akila P, Prashant V, Suma MN, Prashant SN, Chaitra TR. CD163 and its expanding functional repertoire. Clina Chimica Acta. 2012; 413: 669-674.

[4] Alayash Abdu I. Haptoglobin: Old protein with new functions. Clinical Chimiva Acta. 2011; 412: 493-98

[5] Archimandritis A, Theodoropoulos G, Tryphonos M, Germinis A, Tjivras M, Kalos A, Fertakis A. Serum protein markers (Hp, GG, C3 in patients with gastric carcinoma. Hum Hered. 1992; 42 (3): 168-71.

[6] Arredouani MS, Kasran A, Vanoirbeek JA, berger FG, Baumann H, Ceuppens JL. Haptoglobin dampens endotoxin-induced inflammatory effects both in vitro and in vivo. Immunologu. 2005; 114829: 263-71

[7] Awadallah S, Hatoum M. Haptoglobin polymorphism in breast cancer patients from Jordan. Clin Chim Acta. 2004; 341:17-21

[8] Azarov I, He X, Jeffers A, Basu S, Ucer B, Hantgan RR, Levy A, Kim-Shapiro DB. Rate of nitric oxide scavenging by haemoglobin bound to haptoglobin. Nitric Oxide. 2008; 18: 296-302.

[9] Bartel U, Eling D, Gesserick G. Distribution of Hp phenotypes in Gynaecologic tumors. Zentralbl Gynakol 1985; 107 (24) 1492-5

[10] Baumgarten A. Micro method of haptoglobin typing acrylamide gels. Nature 1963; 199: 490-91

[11] Beckman G, Eklund A, Fröhlander N, Stjemberg N. Haptoglobin groups, and lung cancer. Hum Hered 1986; 36: 258-60

[12] Benkmann HG, Hanssen HP, Ovenbeck R, Goedde HW. Distribuition of alpha-1-antitrypsin and haptoglobin phenotypes in bladder cancer patients. Hum Hered.1987; 37: 290-3

[13] Bicho MC, Pereira da Silva A, Matos A, Silva RM, Bicho MD. Sex steroid hormones influence the risk for cervical cancer: Modulation by haptoglobin genetic polymorphism. Cancer Genet Cytogenet. 2009; 191 (2); 85-9

[14] Bicho MC, Pereira da Silva A, Silva RM, Matos A, Fontes G, Bicho MD. Haptoglobin genetic polymorphism interaction with the risk factors for cervix cancer and its precursors lesion. Update on Human Papillomavirus infection and cervical pathology Ed. Joseph Monsonego. Medimond International Proceedings. 2006

[15] Bicho MC. Contribution for the study of biomarkers and cofactors in cervical cancer. PhD Thesis Ed ICBAS Oporto University. 2011. Portugal

[16] Bottini N, Gimelfab A, Gloria-Bottini F, Torre ML, Lucarelli P, Lucarini N. Haptoglobin genotype and natural fertility in humans. Fertil Steril. 1999; 72: 293-6

[17] Bottini N, Gloria-Bottini F, Amante A, Saccucci P Bottini. Genetic polymorphism and Th11/Th2 Orientation. Inter.Arch Allergy immunol. 2005; 138: 328-333

[18] Bowman BH. Haptoglobin: Bowman BH, editor. Hepatic plasma proteins, San Diego: Academic Press. 1993: 159-67

[19] Bowman BH, Kurosky A. Haptoglobin: the evolutionary product of duplication, unequal crossing over and point mutation. Adv Hum. Genet 1982; 12; 189-261

[20] Bresalier RS, Byrd JC, Tessler D, Lebel J, Koomen J, Hawke D, Half E, Liu KF, Mazurek N. A circulating ligand for galectin-3 is a haptoglobin-reated glycoprotein eleved in individuals with colon cancer. Gastroenterology. 2004; 127 (3): 741-8

[21] Campos SP and Baumann H. Insulin is a prominent modulator of the cytokine-stimulated expression of acute-phase plasma protein genes. Mol. Cell. Biol. 1992; 12; 4: 1789-97

[22] Campregher PV, Metze IL, Grotto HZW, Sonati MF. Haptoglobin phenotypes in Brazilian patients with leukemia. J Bras Pet Med Lab. 2004; 40: 307-9

[23] Chen Chao-Bin, Su Yu-chieh, Huang Tze-Ta, Ho Hsu-Chueh, Chang Ya-Ting, Tung Ya-Ting, Lee Wen-Chien. Differentially expressed serum haptoglobin alpha chain isoforms with potential application for diagnosis of head and neck cancer. Clinica Chimica Acta. 2008; 398: 48-52.

[24] Cid MC, Grant DS, Hoffman GS, Auerbach R, Fauci AS, Kleinman HK. Identification of haptoglobin as an angiogenic factor in sera from patients with systemic vasculitis. J Clin Invest. 1993; 91: 977-85

[25] Clerici M, Shearer GM, Clerici E. J Nat cancer Inst. 1998; 90(4): 261-63

[26] Cozzi A, Corsi B, Levi S, Santambrogio P, Biasiotto G, Arosio P. Analysis of the biological functions of H- and L-ferritins in HeLa cells by transfection with siRNAs and cDNAs: Evidence for a proliferative role of L-ferritin. Blood. 2004; 103: 2377-83

[27] Deng R, Lu Z, Chen Y, Zou L, Lu X. Plasma protein analysis of pancreatic cancer by 2-dimensional gel electrophoresis. Pancreas. 2007; 34(3): 310-7

[28] Dimopoulos MA, Germinis A, Savides P, Karayanis A, Fertakis A, Dimopoulos C. Genetic markers in carcinoma of the prostate. Eur Urolo. 1994; 10 (5): 315-6.

[29] Dobryszycka W and Wavas M. Haptoglobin types in ovarian tumors. Neoplasm. 1983; 30: 169-72.

[30] Dunzendorfer U, Ohlenschlager G, Zahradnik HP. 13,14-Dihydro-15-ket prostaglandin F2 alpha and haptoglobin in the serum of patients with urogenital tumors. Onkologie. 1981; 4 (1): 10-16.

[31] EL Ghmati SM, Van Hoeyveld EM, Van Strijp JG, Ceuppens JL, Stevens EA. Identification of haptoglobin as an alternative ligand for CD11b/CD18.J.Immunol. 1996; 156 (7): 2542-52.

[32] Fagoonee S, Gburek J, Hirsch E, Marro S, Moestrup SK, Laurberg JM, Chiristensem EI, Silengo L, Altruda F and Tolosano E. Plasma protein haptoglobin modulate renal iron loading. Am J. of Pathol. 2005; 166: 973-83.

[33] Friedrichs WE, Navarijo-Ashbaugh AL, Bowman BH, Yang F. Expression and inflammatory regulation of haptoglobin gene in adipocytes. Biochem Biophys Res Commun. 1995; 209: 250-256.

[34] Fröhlander N and Stendahl U. Haptoglobin groups in ovarian carcinoma. Hum Hered. 1988; 38: 180-182.

[35] Gast M-C W, van Tinteren H, Bontenbal M, van Hoesel QGGCM, Nooij MA, Rodenhuis S, Span PN, Tjan-Heijnen VCG, de Vries EGE, Harris N, Twisk JWR, Schellens JHM, Beijjnen J. Haptoglobin phenotype is not predictor of recurrence free survival in high-risk primary breast cancer patients. Research article. BMC Cancer. 2008; 8; 389: 1-15.

[36] Germenis A, Babionitakis A, Kaloterakis A, Filotou A, Fertakis A. Group-specific component and haptoglobin phenotypes in multiple myeloma. Hum Hered. 1983; 33: 188-91.

[37] Germinis A, Savides P, Dimopoulos MA, Becopoulos T, Fertakis A, Dimopoulos C. Genetic markers in benign hypertrophy of the prostate. Press Med. 1983; 19; 12 (12): 751-2.

[38] Giannoni E, Chiarugi P, Coozi G. Magnelle L, taddei ML, Fiaschi T, Buricchi F, Raugei G, Ramponi G. Lymphocyte function associated-antigen-1 mediated T cell adhesion is impaired by low molecular weight phosphotyrosine phosphatase-dependent inhibition of FAK activity. J.Biol Chem. 2003; 36763-76.

[39] Giblett ER, The haptoglobin system.Ser Haematol. 1968: 13-20.

[40] Gleeson M. Introdution to the Immune System. In "Immune Function in Sport and Exercise" Ed by Michael Gleeson; Advances in Sport and Exercise Science Series ed by Neil Spurway and Don MacLaren. Churchill Livingstone Elsevier. 2006; 2: 15-43.

[41] Graversen JH, Madsen M, Moestrup SK. CD163: a signal receptor scavenging haptoglobin-haemoglobin complexes from plasma. The Inter J Biochem &Cell Biol. 2002; 34: 309-314.

[42] Gruys E, Toussant MJM, Niewold TA, Koopmans SJ. Acute phase reaction and acute phase proteins. J Zhejiang Univ SCI. 2005; 6B (11): 1045-56.

[43] Guerra A, Monteiro C, Breitenfeld L, Jardim H, Rego C, Siva D, Prata A, Mato SJ, Pereira A, Teixeira SN, Bicho M. Genetic and environmental factors regulating blood pressure in childhood: prospective study from 0 to 3 years. J.Human Hypertension. 1997; 1: 233-238.

[44] Guetta J, Strauss M, Levy NS, Fahoum L, Levy AP. Haptoglobin genotype modulates the balance of Th1/Th2 cytokines produced by macrophages exposed to free haemoglobin. Atherosclerosis. 2007; 191, 48-53.

[45] Gutteridge JMC. The antioxidant activity of haptoglobin towards haemoglobin-stimulated lipid peroxidation. Biochem Biophys Acta. 1987; 917: 219-23.

[46] Harvey S, Kohga S, Sait SN, Markus G, Hurd TC, Martnick M, Geradts J, Saxena R, Gibbs JF. Co-expression of urokinase with haptoglobin in human carcinomas. J.Surg Res. 2009; 152(2): 189-97.

[47] Hudson BL, Sunderland E, Cartwright RA, Benson EA, Smiddy FG, Cartwright SC. Haptoglobin phenotypes in two series of breast cancer patients. Hum Hered. 1982; 32: 219-21.

[48] Jayanthi M, Habibullah CM, Ishaq M, Ali H, Babu PS, Ali MM. Distribution of haptoglobin phenotypes in oesophageal and gastric cancer. J Med Genet. 1989; 26: 172-3.

[49] Kaisho T, Alkira S. Toll-like receptors as adjuvant receptors. Biochem. Biophy. Acta. 2002; 1589: 1-13.

[50] Kaur H, Bhardwaj DN, Shrivastava PK, Sehajal PK, Singh JP, Paul BC. Serum protein polymorphisms in breast cancer. Acta Anthropog. 1984, 8:189-97.

[51] Kendall PA, Saeed SA, Collier HO. Identification of endogenous inhibitor of prostaglandin synthetase with haptoglobin and albumin. Biochem Soc Trans 1979; 7(3): 543-5.

[52] Kuhajda FP, Katumuluwa AI, Pasternack GR. Expression of haptoglobin-related protein and its potencial role as a tumor antigen. PNAS, 1989; 86; 1188-92

[53] Kuhajda FP, Piantadosi S, Pasternack GR. Haptoglobin-related protein (Hpr) epitopes in breast cancer as a predictor of recurrence of the disease. N Engl J Med. 1989; 321: 636-41

[54] Kumar DM, Thota B, Shinde SV, Prasana KV, Hegde AS, Arivazhagan A, Chandramouli BA, Santosh V, Somasundaram K. Proteomic identification of haptoglobin $\alpha2$

as a gliobastoma serum biomarker: implication in cancer cell migration and tumor growth. J Proteome Res. 2010; 5; 9(11): 5557-67.

[55] Langlois MR and Delanghe JR. Biological and clinical significance of haptoglobin in human. Clin Chem. 1996; 42: 1589-600.

[56] Larkin M. Serum Haptoglobin type and cancer. JNCI. 1967; 39: 633-8.

[57] Larsen K, Macleod D, Nihlberg K, Gürcan E, Bjermer L, Marko-Varga G, Westergren-Thorsson. Specific haptoglobin expression in bronchoalveolar lavage during differentiation of circulating fibroblast progenitor cells in mild asthma. J Proteome Res. 2006; 5(6): 1479-83

[58] Lee CC, Lin HY, Hung SK, Li DK, Ho HC, Lee MS, Tung YT, Chou P, Su YC. Haptoglobin genotypes in nasopharyngeal carcinoma. Int J Biol Markers. 2009; 24(1): 32-7

[59] Levy AP, Asleh R, Blum S, Levy NS, Miller-lotan R et al. Haptoglobin: Basic and clinical aspects. Antioxidants & Redox signalling. 2010; 12; 2: 293-304

[60] Linke RP. Tying and subtyping of haptoglobin from native serum using disc gel electrophoresis in alkaline buffer, application to routing screening. Anal Biochem. 1984; 141: 55-61

[61] Liu XH, Kirschenbaum A, Lu M, Yao S, Dosoret A, Holland JF, Levine AC. Prostaglandin E2 induces hypoxia-inducible factor-1α stabilization and nuclear localization in a human prostate cancer cell line. J.Biol Chem. 2002; 277 (51): 5081-6.

[62] Lu JY, Wu ZQ, Tan LN, Chen J, Xiang YP, Zuo CX, Huang JH, Jiang XZ. mRNA and protein expression of haptoglobina in lesion of condiloma acuminatum. Zhong Nan Da Xue Bao Yi Xue Ban. 2007; 32 (6): 1020-5.

[63] Lucey DR, Clerici M, e Shearer GM.Type 1 and Type 2 Cytokine Dysregulation in Human Infectious Neoplastic and Inflammatory Diseases. Clinical Microbiology Reviews. 1996: 532-562.

[64] Maeda N, Yang F, Barnett DR, Bowman BH, Smithies O. Duplication within the haptoglobin Hp2 gene. Nature. 1984; 309; 131-5.

[65] Mahmud SM, Koushik A, Duarte E, Costa J, Fontes J, Bicho M, Coutlée F, Franco E.Haptoglobin fenotype and risk of cervical neoplasia: case-control study. Clin.Chem. Acta. 2007; 385: 67-72.

[66] Mavondo GA, Mangemna Z, Kasvosve I. Haptoglobin polymorphism is not associated with prostate cancer in blacks. Clinica Chimica Acta. 2012; 413: 334-336

[67] Mihailović M, Dinić S, Uskoković A, Petrović M, Grigorov I, Poznanović G, Ivanović-Matić S, Bogojević D. Acute-phase related binding ability of p53 for the hormone response element of the haptoglobin gene in adult rats. Cell Biol Int. 2005; 29(11): 968-70.

[68] Milunicova A, Jandova A, Skoda A. Serum haptoglobin type in females with genital cancer. J N Cancer Inst. 1969; 42: 749-51.

[69] Mitchell RJ, Carzino R, Janardhana V. Association between the two serum proteins haptoglobin and transferrin and leukemia. Hum Hered. 1988; 38: 144-50.

[70] Miyoshi E, Nakkano M. Fucosylated haptoglobin is a novel marker for pancreatic cancer: detailed analyses of oligosaccharide structures. Proteomics. 2008; 8 (16): 3257-62

[71] Moestrup SK, Møller HJ. CD163: A regulated haemoglobin scavenger receptor with a role in the anti-inflammatory response. Ann Med. 2004; 36: 347-54.

[72] Nakano M, Nakagawa T, Ito T, Kitada T, Hijioka T, Kasahara A, Tajiri M, Wada Y, Taniguchi N, Miyoshi E. Site-specific analysis of N-glycans on haptoglobin in sera of patients with pancreatic cancer: a novel approach for the development of tumor markers. Int J Cancer. 2008; 15; 122(10): 2301-9

[73] Nascimento CO, Hunter L and Trayhurn P. Regulation of haptoglobin gene expression in 3T3-L1 adipocytes by cytokines, catecholamines, and PPARγ. Biochem Biophys Res Commun. 2004; 313: 702-708.

[74] Nevo S and Tatarsky I. Serum haptoglobin types and leukemia. Hum Hered. 1986; 73: 240-44

[75] Nielsen MJ, Møller HJ, Moestrup SK. Hemoglobin and heme scavenger receptors. Antioxidants & Redox Signaling. 2010; 12; 2: 261-273

[76] Nielson MJ, Petersen SV, Jacobsen C, Oxvig C, Rees D, Møller HJ, Moestrup SK. Haptoglobin-related protein is a high-affinity hemoglobin-binding plasma protein. Blood. 2006; 108: 2846-49

[77] Oh M-K, Parh H-J, Kim N-H, Park S-J, In Y-P, In Sk. Hypoxia-inducible factor-1α enhances haptoglobin gene expression by improving binding of STAT3 to the promoter. JBC. 2011; 286; 11: 8857-65

[78] Olson GE, Winfrey VP, Matrisian PE, Melner MH, Hoffman LH. Specific expression of haptoglobin mRNA in implantation-stage rabbit uterine epithelium. J. Endocrinol. 1997; 152: 69-80

[79] Palayoor ST, Tofilon PJ, Coleman CN. Ibuprofen-mediated reduction of hypoxia – inducible factors HIF-1α and HIF-2 α in prostate cancer cells. Clinical Cancer Research. 2003; 9: 3150-7

[80] Park SJ, Baek SH, Oh Mk, Chui SH, Park EH, Kin NH, Shin Jc, Kim IS. Enhancement of angiogenic and vasculogenic potential of endothelial progenitor cells by haptoglobin. FEBS Lett. 2009; 583(19): 3235-40.

[81] Quaye IK, Agbolosu K, Ibrahim M, Bannerman-Williams P. Haptoglobin phenotypes in cervical: decreased risk for Hp2-2 individuals. Clinica Chimica Acta. 2009; 403: 267-68.

[82] Raynes JG, Ealing S, McAdam KP. Acute-phase protein synthesis in human hepatoma cells: Differential regulation of serum amyloid A (SAA) and haptoglobin by interleukin-1 and interleukin-6. Clin Exp Immunol. 1991; 83: 488-91

[83] Ron D, Brasier AR, and Haberner JF. Transcriptional regulation of hepatic angiotensinogen gene expression by the acute-phase response. Molecular and Cellular Endocrinology. 1990; 74: C97-C104.

[84] Sadrzadeh SMH and Bozorgmehr J. Haptoglobin phenotypes in health and disorders. Am J Clin Pathol (reviews). 2004; 121(1): S97-S104

[85] Sadrzadeh SMH, Graf E, Panter SS, Hallaway PE, Eaton JW. Hemoglobin – A biologic Fenton reagent. J.Biol Chem. 1984; 259: 14354-6

[86] Saeed SA, Ahmad N, Ahmed S. Dual inhibition of cyclooxygenase and lipoxigenase by human haptoglobin: Its polymorphism and relation to hemoglobin binding. Biochem Biophys Res Commun. 2007; 353: 915- 920

[87] Saito S, Murayama Y, Pan Y, Taima T, Fujimura T, Murayama K, Sadilek M, Egawa S, Ueno S, Ito A, Ishidoya S, Nakagawa H, Kato M, Satoh M, Endoh M, Arai Y. Haptoglobin-beta chain defined by monoclonal antibody RM2 as a novel serum marker for prostate cancer. Inter J Cancer. 2008; 123(3) : 633-40

[88] Sanchez DJ, Armstrong L, Aguilar R, Adrian GS, Haro L, Martinez AO. Haptoglobin gene expression in human glioblastoma cell lines. Neurosci Lett. 2001; 11; 303(3): 181-4

[89] Sharpe-Timms KL, Zimmer RL, Ricke EA, Piva M. Horowitz GM. Endometriotic haptoglobin binds to peritoneal macrophages and alters their function in women with endometriosis. Fertility and Stetirility. 2002; 78 (4): 810-118

[90] Shaw JLV, Smith CR, Diamandis EP. Proteomic analysis of human cervico-vaginal fluid.J.of Proteome Research 2007, 6, 2859-2865

[91] Smithies O. Zone electrophoresis in starch gels group variation in the serum proteins of normal human adults. Biochem J. 1955; 61: 628-641

[92] Speeckaert R, Brochez L, Lambert J, Van Geel N, Speeckaert MM, Claeys LR, Langlois M, Van Laer C, Peeters P, Delanghe JR. The haptoglobin phenotype influences the risk of cutaneous squamous cell carcinoma in kidney transplant patients. J.Eur Acad Dermatol Venereol. 2012; 26(5): 566-71.

[93] Speeckaert R, Colebunders B, Boelaert JR, Brochez L, Van Acker J, Van Wanzeele F, Hemmer R, Speeckaert MM, Verhofstede C, De Buyzere M, Arendt V, Plum J, De-

langhe JR. Association of haptoglobin phenotypes with the development of Kaposi's sarcoma in HIV patients. Arch Dermatol Res. 2011; 303(10): 763-9.

[94] Speeckaert R, Speeckaert MM, Padalko E, Claeys LR, Delanghe JR. The haptoglobin phenotype is associated with the Epstein-Barr virus antibody. Clin Chem Lab Med. 2009; 47(7): 826-8

[95] Theilgaard-Mönch K, Jacobsen LC, Nielsen MJ, Rasmussen T et al. Haptoglobin is synthesized during granulocyte differentiation, stored in specific granules, and released by neutrophils in response to activation. Blood. 2006; 108: 353-61.

[96] Theodoropoulos G, Archimandritis A, Germinis A, Malamas N, Tjivras M, Fertakis A. Serum protein markers (Hp, GG, C3 in patients with colon cancer. Hum Hered. 1993; 43 (1): 66-8

[97] Touitou Y, Proust J, Carayon A, Klinger E, Nakache JP, Huard D, Sachet A. Plasma ferritin in old age. Influence of biological and pathological factors in a large elderly population. Clinica Chimica Acta. 1985; 149: 37-45.

[98] Trautwein C, Böker K, Mannus MP. Hepatocyte and imune system: acute phase reaction as a contribution to early defence mechanisms. Gut. 1994; 35: 1163-66.

[99] Tsamantains C, Delinassios JG, Kottaridis S, Christodoulou C. Haptoglobin types in breast carcinoma. J, Hum Hered. 1980; 30 (1): 44-5.

[100] Vallelian F, Schaer CA. Kaempfer T, Gehrig P, Duerst E, Schoedon G, Schaer D. Glucorticoid treatment skews human monocyte differentiation into a haemoglobin-clearance phenotype with enhance heme-iron recycling and antioxidant capacity. Blood. 2010; 116; 24: 5347-56.

[101] Van Vlierberghe H, Langlois M, Delanghe J. Haptoglobin Polymorphism and iron homeostasis in health and disease, Clinica Chimica Acta. 2004; 345: 35-42

[102] Vlierberghe HV, Langlois M, Delanghe. Haptoglobin polymorphisms and iron homeostasis in health and in disease. Clinica Chimica Acta. 2004; 345: 35-42.

[103] Wang H, Gao XH, Wang YK, Li P, He CD, Xie Y, Chen HD. Expression of haptoglobin in human keratinocytes and langerhans cells. Br. J.Dermatol. 2005; 153 (5): 894-899.

[104] Weinberg ED. Iron withholding: a defence against viral infections. Biometais. 1996; 9 (4): 393-9.

[105] Wen WN. Methemoglobin is a suplement for in vitro culture of human nasopharyngeal epithelial cells transformed by human papillomavirus types 16 DNA. In Vitro Cell Dev Biol Anim. 2001; 37(10): 668-75.

[106] Wenger RH, Rolfs A, Marti HH, Bauer C, Gassmann M. Hypoxia, a novel inducer of acute phase gene expression in a human hepatoma cell line. J Biol Chem. 1995; 17; 270(46): 27865-70

[107] Wicher KB, Fries E. Convergent evolution of human and bovine haptoglobin: partial duplication of the genes. L Mol Evol. 2007; 65: 373-79.

[108] Wobeto VPA, Zaccariotto TR and Sonati MF. Polymorphism of human haptoglobin and its clinical impotance. Genetics and Molecular Biology. 2008; 31; 3: 602-20.

[109] XiaLi-xin, Xiao Ting, Chen Hong-duo, Li Ping, Wang Ya-kun, Wang He. Regulation of haptoglobin expression in a human keratinocyte cell line HaCaT by inflammatory cytokines and dexamethasone. Chin Med J. 2008; 121(8): 730-34.

[110] Xie Y, Li Y, Zhang Q, Stiller MJ, Albert Wang CL, Wayne Streilein J. Haptoglobin is a natural regulator of Langerhans cell function in the skin. J. Dermat Science. 2000; 24: 25-37.

[111] Yang F, Ghio AJ, Herbert DC, Weaker FJ, Waltwer CA and Coalson JJ. Pulmonary expression of the human haptoglobin gene. Am J. Respir Cell Mol. Biol. 2000; 23: 277-82.

[112] Ye YN, Liu ESL, Shin VY, Wu WKK, Cho CH. The modulating role of nuclear factor-kB in the action of α-7-nicotinic acetylcholine receptor and cross-talk between 5-lipoxygenase and cycloxygenase-2 in colon cancer growth induced by 4-(N-methyl-N-nitrosamino)-1-(3-pyridyl)-1-butanone. J Pharmacol Exp Therap (JPET). 2004; 311(1): 123-30.

[113] Ye YN, Wu WKK, Shin VY, Cho CH. A mechanistic study of colon cancer growth promoted by cigarette smoke extract. European J Pharmacol. 2005; 519: 52-7.

[114] Zur Hausen H. Papillomaviruses and cancer: From basic studies to clinical application. Nature Reviews. May 2002 V2 342-50.

Chapter 4

Role of SAA in Promoting Endothelial Activation: Inhibition by High-Density Lipoprotein

Xiaosuo Wang, Xiaoping Cai,
Saul Benedict Freedman and Paul K. Witting

Additional information is available at the end of the chapter

http://dx.doi.org/10.5772/56047

1. Introduction

Serum amyloid A (SAA) is a multi-gene family consisting of highly conserved protein sequences that are known to cluster on chromosome 11 in humans [1] and chromosome 7 in mice [2]. The acute-phase proteins SAA1 and SAA2 (mass of ~12 kDa, 104 amino acids) share > 93% identity in primary sequence structure, are secreted predominantly by hepatocytes and are induced by a broad spectrum of inflammatory cytokines [3]. Extra-hepatic production of acute-phase SAA occurs in many organs and tissues of body including vascular smooth muscle cells and endothelial cells (EC) that are also capable of secreting SAA [4, 5]. By contrast, SAA4 is a glycosylated form that is constitutively produced in a wide range of (histologically) normal tissues and cells [6]. The final isoform, SAA3, is a pseudogene that is not transcribed in humans [1]. In rodents, SAA3 is a functional protein that is expressed in extra-hepatic cells, such as macrophages and adipocytes in response to prolactin or lipolysaccaride (LPS) stimuli thereby, contributing to local inflammation in adipose tissues [7, 8].

Rapid production of SAA in response to the host inflammatory reaction results in plasma levels increasing up to 1,000-fold under some conditions [9]. This marked increase in circulating SAA is linked to the induction of inflammatory cascades that are characterized by local vascular, systemic and multi-organ responses [10, 11]. A wealth of epidemiological and biological research suggests that SAA is also associated with chronic inflammatory conditions such as cardiovascular diseases (CVD) and atherogenesis [12-14]. For example, significantly elevated levels of SAA are evident at different stages of atherosclerosis [15, 16], which, to some extent, echoes a sustained acute-phase response leading to the chronic production of SAA. In fact, SAA is proposed as a potential regulator of inflammation and endothelial dysfunction, implicating adverse outcomes that complicate CVD [4]. SAA is also synthesized in extrahepatic tissues and involved in human carcinoma growth and metastases suggesting SAA could participate in tumor development [14] through stimulating pro-angiogenic factors.

The association of circulating SAA with high-density lipoprotein (HDL) is well described with the majority of SAA incorporated as an HDL apolipoprotein [17]. Recent research has focused on the influence of SAA on HDL structure and function (*i.e.*, anti-inflammatory and antioxidant activities of the lipoprotein), including the impact of SAA on HDL's role in reverse cholesterol transport.

2. General pro-inflammatory/pro-thrombotic responses to SAA

SAA may represent a useful clinical marker of acute and chronic inflammation [18]. Similar to the biomarker C-reactive protein (CRP), SAA increases in the blood of patients with various inflammatory conditions. A growing body of research supports the notion that SAA is a potent and rapid inducer of cytokines, monocyte tissue factor (TF) and tumor necrosis factor-α (TNF-α) in human peripheral blood mononuclear cells (PBMC) and THP-1 monocytoid cells within a short period of exposure [19-22]. Initially, this SAA-stimulated cell activation is limited to the local sites of the inflammation. However, upon activation of macrophages, a range of primary inflammatory mediators are released, the most important of which are members of the IL-1 and TNF families of cytokines. These in turn cause the release of secondary cytokines and chemokines (*e.g*, IL-6, IL-8 and MCP-1) from local stromal cells [4, 23]. The chemotactic activities of these chemokines recruit leukocytes such as neutrophils to the inflammatory site, where they in turn provoke a sustained pro-inflammatory cascade that involves local production and release of other cytokines [10,23].

As indicated, SAA stimulation of PMBCs causes a marked increase in the secretion of cytokines including IL-1B, MCP-1, IL-6, IL-8, IL-10, GM-CSF, TNF and MIP-1α with reports of up to 25,000-fold increase compared to baseline levels measured in isolated monocytes / macrophages and lymphocytes [20]. In addition, SAA strongly induces the potent pro-coagulant protein TF, and this activity manifests as an inflammatory-associated thrombosis that also impairs endothelial function. The release of SAA into the circulation in subjects with established coronary artery disease (CAD) may play a role in promoting cardiovascular events since SAA stimulates the expression of TF and TNF in isolated PBMCs [20, 21]. Given the nature of TNF itself as a mediator of inflammatory and its co-localization to atherosclerotic lesions, and TF as a potent pro-coagulating factor, then the concomitant release of these factors is likely to represent a central feature in the pathogenesis and clinical complications associated with developing CAD.

An increase in the circulating levels of SAA may enhance TF expression [24]. Studies have demonstrated that TF binds instantly to TF activated factor VII (FVIIa) yielding a complex that serves as a fuse to facilitate blood coagulation by generating thrombin [24]. Furthermore, activated FVIIa stimulates TF provoked factor VII, IX and X, a secondary cascade that ultimately leads to more thrombin formation [24, 25]. In addition to a direct stimulating effect on TF, SAA also acts on vascular EC to modulate TF pathway inhibitors through a mechanism involving mitogen-activated protein kinase (MAPK) and the transcription factor, nuclear factor kappa beta (Nfκβ) [25]. Activation of MAPK and Nfκβ) are central to the induction of cytokines by SAA [26, 27].

3. Response of endothelial cells to SAA

A functional endothelium is vital to the maintenance of vascular homeostasis [28]. The primary function of the vascular endothelium is to act as a barrier that regulates vascular permeability to plasma constituents and inhibits platelet and leukocyte adhesion and aggregation as well as infiltration, and finally, regulates thrombosis [29]. Thus the vascular EC is crucial for maintaining vascular tone, fluidity, coagulation, and inflammatory responses [30]. Under normal physiological conditions, vascular homeostasis is controlled by potent mediators such as nitric oxide (NO), prostacyclin-2 and endothelin-1 as well as local angiotensin II activity [31].

Endothelial dysfunction occurs before the appearance of the first morphological signs of atherosclerosis and is a precursor of atherogenesis [32], therefore endothelial dysfunctional can predict the extent of CVD [33]. Redox regulation of intracellular signaling has been implicated as a factor that impacts on endothelial activation [34]. For example, redox modulation of endothelial nitric oxide synthase (eNOS) gene expression, transport of the active dimeric form of eNOS to the cell membrane by lipid rafts and/or eNOS activity can in turn have downstream effects on NO bioavailability and signaling [35]. Decreases in eNOS activity may contribute to endothelial dysfunction by impairing endothelium-dependent vasorelaxation. Alternatively, decreased production of NO can activate other mediators that play important roles in atherogenesis [Reviewed in 36, 37].

Once the balance of vascular homeostasis is compromised the vascular endothelium undergoes a phenotypic change associated with increased expression of intracellular adhesion molecule-1 (ICAM-1), vascular cell adhesion molecule-1 (VCAM-1), E-selectin, and pro-inflammatory cytokines such as TNF-α, IL-1, IL-6, IFN-γ together with pro-thrombotic factors. Under these conditions the formation of reactive oxygen species (ROS) is increased and this can impact on vascular tone that is susceptible to oxidative stress via a range of mechanisms [29, 31]. For example, the stability of eNOS and production of NO is directly affected by ROS. Indeed, oxidative events have featured in many studies of impaired NO bioactivity [38] and endothelial dysfunction, which in turn impacts on other cardiovascular risk factors such as hypertension [39], diabetes [40] and rheumatic autoimmune diseases [32].

Studies have shown that SAA also promotes both monocyte chemotaxis and adhesion to the vascular endothelium [5, 41], thereby regulating the recruitment of leukocytes to the inflamed endothelium [42]. During this process SAA promotes the production of other pro-inflammatory cytokines and chemotactic molecules, which cause endothelial dysfunction and ultimately lead to atherosclerosis and other related CAD. In support of this idea it is found that SAA co-localizes within microtubules of human coronary artery EC (HCAEC) [43]. Previous work from our group [44] has confirmed that SAA stimulates EC production of TF and Nfκβ gene expression as well as cytokines such as IL-6, IL-8, and MCP-1 that in turn impair NO bioactivity

[44]. For example, exposure of isolated thoracic aortic vessels to SAA (1-25 μg/mL) decreases vascular relaxation in response to the endothelium-dependent vaso-dilator acetylcholine (ACh) (Fig. 1A), whereas endothelium-independent vaso-relaxation to s-nitrosopenicillamine (SNP) remained unaffected by SAA (Fig. 1B). A similar study by Wang and co-workers has reported that clinically relevant concentrations of SAA causes endothelial dysfunction in both porcine coronary arteries and HCAEC by down regulation of eNOS, activation of JNK and ERK1/2 as well as Nfκβ [45]. This mechanism is consistent with a study indicating that inhibitors of MAPK and Nfκβ markedly decreased SAA-stimulated pro-inflammatory cytokines secretion from HEK293 cells [27]. Taken together these combined data demonstrate that SAA enhances stimulates ROS production in cultured EC [47].

Reactive species such as superoxide radical anion ($O_2^{\bullet-}$), lipid (per)oxidation products and the potent oxidizing agent peroxynitrite are all implicated in endothelial activation and impaired NO signaling. Therefore, SAA-stimulation of ROS production is a possible mechanism to explain impaired endothelial function [44, 48]. In agreement with this hypothesis, exposure of cultured EC to SAA (added at a final concentration of 10 μg/mL) reduces NO accumulation in HCAEC stimulated with ACh, whereas human serum albumin (HSA), that is not known to affect EC production of NO, has no effect (Fig. 2). Interestingly, pre-incubating HCAEC with HDL (50 - 200 μg/mL) before addition of SAA restores NO accumulation in response to ACh, and this is dependent on the dose of HDL (Fig. 2) [44]. Moreover, these data indicate that the ratio of SAA-to-HDL might be critical to assessing SAA's effect on the vascular endothelium.

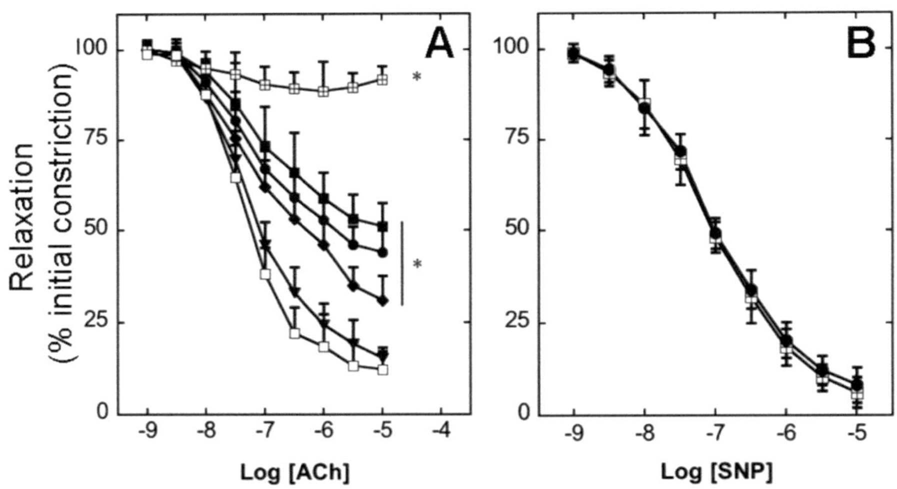

Figure 1. SAA inhibits endothelium-dependent, but not endothelium-independent, relaxation. Aortic rings were incubated with SAA at 1 (inverted triangles), 5 (diamonds), 10 (circles), or 25 μg/mL (solid squares); the soluble guanylate cyclase inhibitor ODQ [46] (used as a positive control, hatched square); or vehicle (control, open squares) for 4 h at 37 °C. Rings were washed and constricted with phenylephrine and then dilated by adding (A) ACh or (B) SNP at the concentrations indicated. Data represent means ± SD (n=6 rings from independent animals except for vessels exposed to 25 μg/mL SAA, n=5 rings from independent animals). *Different to the control in the absence of SAA; $P < 0.05$. The figure was reprinted from Ref [44] with permission from the Publisher.

http://dx.doi.org/10.5772/56047

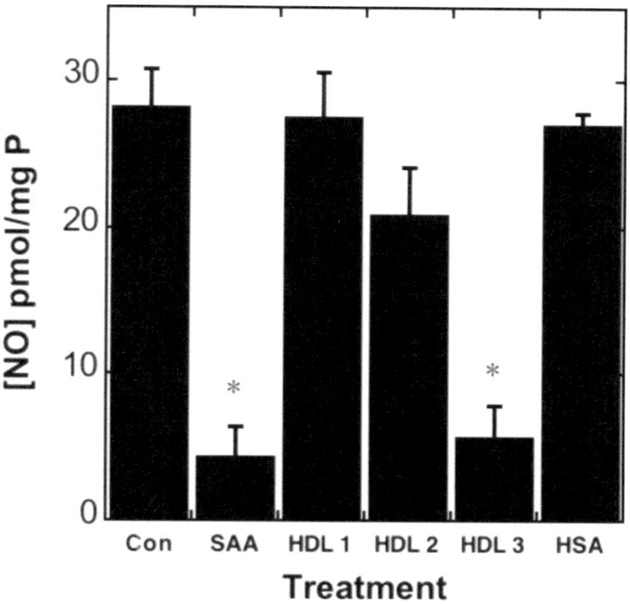

Figure 2. SAA decreased acetylcholine-induced NO accumulation in HCAEC. HCAECs were pretreated in serum-free-medium containing vehicle (control), SAA (10 µg/mL), or human serum albumin (HSA; 1 mg/mL). After 4 h cells were harvested, resuspended in HPSS (~4×106 cells/mL) containing 100 µM Arginine and stimulated with 1 µM ACh. Changes in NO evolution were monitored with an NO electrode. Freshly isolated HDL (50 - 200 µg/mL) added 30 min before incubation with SAA inhibited the action of the acute phase protein. Total nitrite was determined in the medium after incubation with nitrate reductase / NADPH. HDL1, 50; HDL2, 100; and HDL3, 200 µg/mL in protein, respectively. Data represent n=3 HCAEC preparations. Figure reprinted from Ref [44] with permission from the publisher.

Previous studies have identified NADPH-oxidase as a significant source of $O_2^{\bullet-}$ in various cell types, in addition to other potential sources such as uncoupled eNOS, xanthine oxidase, mitochondria and cytochrome p450 [38, 47, 49, 50]. The data shown in Fig 3 demonstrate an enhanced yield of $O_2^{\bullet-}$ after stimulation of cultured HCAEC with added SAA. This increase is inhibited by the pharmacological agents diphenyliodonium (DPI) and apocynin (that target NADPH oxidase) or polyethylene glycated SOD-1-conjugate (PEG-SOD) that binds to the cells and promotes $O_2^{\bullet-}$ dismutation [51]. Pre-incubation of cells with HDL (final concentrations 200 and 100, but not 50 µg/mL) reversed SAA-induced responses, again indicating that the SAA-to-HDL ratio is a determinant of SAA-mediated endothelial dysfunction [44].

Other ROS derived from the uncontrolled production of $O_2^{\bullet-}$, such as hydrogen peroxide (H_2O_2) and hydroxyl radical (.OH) can also affect endothelium-dependent contractile responses [52]. For example H_2O_2 can promote vascular constriction [53] and its ability to readily cross cell membranes underlies its ability to stimulate matrix metalloproteases (MMP) in the vascular wall [54]. Another example of $O_2^{\bullet-}$-derived ROS is.OH that is implicated in endothelial dysfunction associated with diabetes [55]. Therefore, exposure of the vascular endothelium to SAA can lead to uncontrolled production of multiple ROS that impact on EC function.

Mounting evidence suggests that ROS are key mediators of vascular inflammation and atherosclerosis [45, 56]. The documented ability of SAA to initiate the production and release of pro-inflammatory cytokines is further supplemented by studies that show SAA can propagate ROS production in rabbit aortic EC [48].

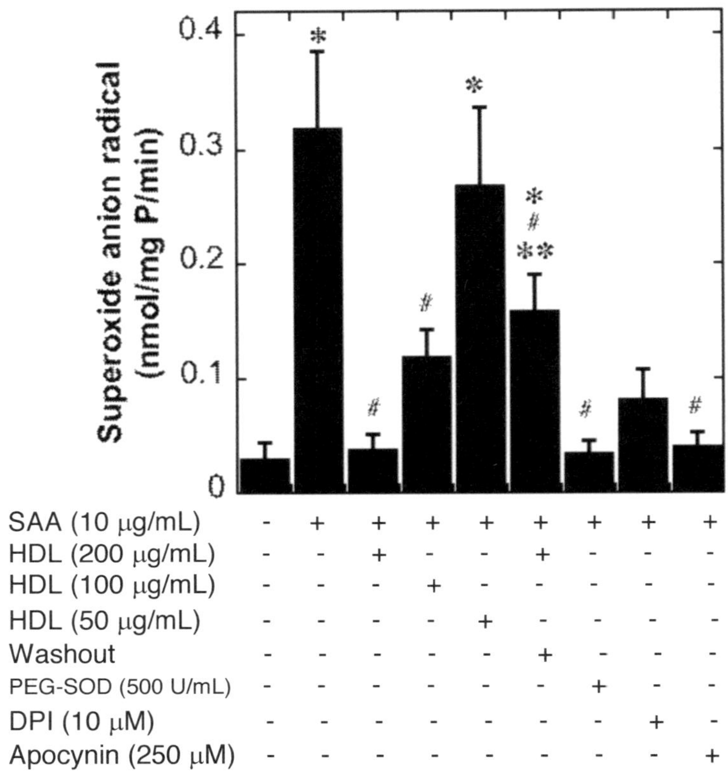

Figure 3. Increased $O_2^{\bullet-}$ production in SAA-stimulated HCAEC. HCAEC (1–2 ×10[6] cells) were treated with 2 μM acetylated ferric cytochrome *c*, SAA (10 μg/mL) was added, and PEG-SOD-inhibitable ferric cytochrome *c* reduction was monitored at 550 nm. Other HCAEC were incubated with 200, 100, or 50 μg HDL/mL for 30 min, then HDL was left in the well or was thoroughly washed out before SAA addition. Other cells were pre-incubated with 10 μM DPI or 250 μM apocynin before SAA stimulation. Data represent means ± SD; n=4 experiments. * Different to unstimulated cells; P<0.05. # Different to HCAEC treated with SAA; P < 0.05. ** Different to the corresponding cells with HDL present; P<0.05. Data represent n=3 experiments. Figure derived from Ref [44] with permission from the Publisher.

Uncontrolled ROS production coupled with impaired antioxidant enzyme activity such as SOD, catalase and glutathione peroxidase (GPx) [57], may also contribute to SAA-mediated EC activation. Further studies implicate P38, JNK/Erk and angiotension II pathways in the deterioration of endothelial function [58, 59]. Overall, the underlying mechanisms implicated in SAA-mediated endothelial dysfunction are multifactorial and include the damage to the NO/eNOS system [45]; enhanced $O_2^{\bullet-}$ production in response to ACh [44], increases in Arg-1 expression [44], and the deficiency of antioxidant systems [53, 57, 60]. Regulation of argi-

http://dx.doi.org/10.5772/56047

nase-1/2 is linked to the up-stream expression of TNF that is induced by SAA and itself promotes vascular dysfunction by decreasesing the pool of substrate available to eNOS [61].

4. SAA and atherosclerosis

Atherosclerosis may be considered as a chronic inflammatory disease [38]. Circulating SAA levels increase in subjects with CAD and changes with the disease severity [4, 62-65]. Levels of SAA also increase in conditions subject to increased cardiovascular risk, such as obesity [62], diabetes [66, 67], rheumatoid arthritis (RA) [68, 69] and angiographically demonstrable CAD [65]. Although this accumulated supporting evidence is mainly observational, the correlative data have provided the basis of a link between SAA and chronic inflammatory processes associated with atherogenesis.

In the artery wall, various inflammatory cell types are recruited and this may be attributed by SAA's chemo-attractant activity [16]. The stimulation of vascular EC to promote the production of TF and TNF-α, combined with the SAA-induced accumulation of adherent monocytes / macrophages, particularly within lymphocyte-rich areas of vascular plaque, may trigger a focal TF response in addition to SAA action on circulating monocytes, thereby contributing to the highly pro-thrombotic properties of the lipid-rich core within atherosclerotic lesions. Subsequent expression of matrix degrading enzymes will result in plaque instability [21]. Potentially, reoccurring acute inflammation will give rise to cyclical increases in circulating SAA that may incite monocyte adhesion and chemotaxis to the artery wall leading to altered barrier function (*i.e.*, endothelial dysfunction) and an increase in lipid content in the sub-endothelial space [12]. At this point, SAA associated HDL may impact on lipid metabolism and possibly reverse cholesterol transportation in the developing lesion through an intensified affinity to macrophages within the atheroma [70]. The retention of SAA-containing HDL in the arterial wall may be promoted due to SAA's ability to strongly bind to vascular proteoglycans [71, 72]. Increased resident time for SAA in the vascular wall may conceivably stimulate the formation of macrophage foam cells implicating SAA in different stages of atherogenesis [38].

Therefore, in addition to accumulating pro-atherogeneic LDL [73] in the arterial wall, the presence of both SAA-associated HDL and oxidized HDL in close proximity to macrophage scavenger receptors may act in concert to potentiate atherogenesis [73-76]. In support of this idea levels of SAA, but not cholesterol, predict lesion area in cholesterol-fed rabbits [77], suggesting a critical role for SAA in the early stages of lesion development. It is also found that SAA deposition in the vessel wall is present at all stages of atherosclerosis [12, 16]. These chronically elevated SAA concentrations in the arterial wall are commonly associated with the pathogenesis of secondary amyloidosis [78] where SAA retains its ability to induce cytokine and chemokine production, matrix-degrading enzymes, such as collagenases and MMP, and interfere with platelet function [78]. Not surprisingly, SAA is co-located with apolipoprotein A-I (apoA-I) in the vascular wall of patients with peripheral atherosclerosis, particularly in the arterial intima [79], an observation confirmed by presence of co-localization of SAA with both apoA-I and proteoglycans in atherosclerotic lesions [80]. Interestingly, SAA is also present within different compartments of HCAEC such as cytoskeletal filaments including microtubules, inside the nucleus and within nanotubules [43]. The expression of SAA in these compartments may favor the progression of atherosclerosis in the vascular wall.

5. Over-expression of SAA in apolipoportein E deficient mice

The apolipoprotein E-deficient (apoE$^{-/-}$) mouse is widely employed as an animal model of atherosclerosis because of its propensity to develop atherosclerotic lesions [81-83]. A growing body of research supports the idea that SAA can initiate endothelial dysfunction. For example, construction of SAA lentivirus in apoE$^{-/-}$ mice stimulates pro-atherogenic changes in the vessel wall [13]. Furthermore, elevated plasma levels of SAA are detected in an apoE$^{-/-}$ model of obesity that exhibits accelerated atherosclerosis [84].

Interestingly, high levels of SAA are found to be associated with both HDL and LDL in mice fed with a high-fat diet. The later is primarily localized with apoB-containing lipoproteins and biglycan in the vascular wall [84]. Similarly, the use of viral vectors to increase SAA levels in apoE$^{-/-}$ mice result in substantially enhanced plasma levels of IL-6 and TNF-α and increased macrophage infiltration into the sub-endothelial space of early developing vascular lesions [13]. Over-expression of SAA also causes marked increase in the expression of MCP-1 and VCAM-1 in HAEC, thus providing direct evidence that chronic elevation of SAA in the vasculature enhances the progression of atherosclerosis in apoE$^{-/-}$ mice [13]. However, in contrast with this idea, extravascular inflammatory stimuli (*i.e.*, croton oil-induced skin inflammation, *aspergillus fumigatus* antigen-induced allergic lung disease and *A.fumigatus* antigen-induced peritonitis), which also stimulates an increase in circulating SAA levels and has no effect on the progression of atherosclerosis in the same mouse model [85]: the gender of mice employed in these two studies differed and this may be important to the study outcome [86]. Interestingly, the latter model likely elicits multiple inflammatory and antioxidant pathways independent of SAA and this may explain at least in part the differences in lesion size reported.

6. Regulation of endothelial function by HDL bound SAA

One of the principal roles of SAA is its association with HDL and the subsequent modulation of the metabolic properties of HDL. In general, SAA is an apolipoprotein largely associated with HDL_3 (density 1.125–1.21 g/mL) in plasma where it can displace apoA-1 if in sufficiently high concentration in the circulating blood [87-89]: apoA-1 is the major protein responsible for the bioactivities associated with anti-atherogenic HDL [90]. Displacement of apoA-I by SAA results in substantial altered metabolic properties of its main physiological carrier. These changes in the apolipoprotein moieties may transform an originally anti-atherogenic into a pro-atherogenic lipoprotein particle [88], although this is yet to be corroborated by other

http://dx.doi.org/10.5772/56047

independent researchers and further studies are warranted to establish this hypothesis. Nevertheless, factors that affect remodeling of HDL are complex due to putative roles of both apoA-1 and SAA.

A recent HDL proteome study confirmed that protein compositions of HDL from acute coronary syndrome (ACS) patients are shifted to a pro-inflammatory profile that co-incidentally show increased circulating SAA [91]. Similarly, studies involving end-stage renal disease (ESRD) patients, indicate that SAA enriched HDL has reduced anti-inflammatory capacity compared to normal HDL [92, 93]. Such SAA-enriched HDL exerts lower anti-inflammatory properties partly due to enhanced binding capacity of SAA-containing HDL to macrophages [94] and proteoglycans [71] relative to native HDL. Furthermore, SAA impedes HDL's hepatocytic affinity and occurs concomitantly with a decrease in apoA-1 content in SAA - containing HDL [94, 95]. The decrease in HDL apoA-1 may be related to the prevention of apoA-I lipidation caused by SAA-elicited inflammation, resulting in an overall decrease in nascent HDL formation [96-99].

However not all studies support a role for SAA in altering HDL function. Increasing the expression of SAA1 or SAA4 (23 -72 mg/dL) in transgenic mice do not significantly alter apoA-I or HDL cholesterol or affect lipoprotein profiles compared with the wild-type [6]. In other studies, adenoviral vector mediated over expression of SAA in ApoAI$^{-/-}$ mice is unable to substitute for apoA-I in HDL particle formation [100]. Interestingly, in SAA deficient mice (dual SAA-1/2 gene deletion), increased size of HDL is found in relation to surface phospholipids, not proteins. Total HDL levels and apoA-I clearance are resistant to change during inflammation [89, 101].

The proportion of SAA incorporating into HDL as an apolipoprotein may impact on the function of this lipoprotein. A recent perspective review on SAA by Kisilevsky *et al* [99] has detailed estimates of molar ratios between HDL and SAA in different clinical settings (Table 1). In the setting of developing CAD, ~10% of circulating HDL contains SAA, whereas in an acute inflammatory response every HDL particle contains at lease one SAA. By contrast in a normal physiological setting few HDL particles contain SAA [99]. It is estimated that when SAA constitutes 10-20% or more of total HDL protein, HDL binding capacity to PBMC and EC is increased relative to native HDL [95].

Furthermore, 8-10% incorporation of SAA in total HDL protein causes slight increases in the release of pro-inflammatory cytokines from adipocytes [102]. Outcomes from cell culture studies suggest that reduction of cholesterol efflux by SAA bound HDL is not pronounced unless SAA constitutes more than 50% of the total HDL protein [17]. A similar study confirms that impaired ABCG1-dependent efflux by HDL is independent of SAA during inflammation, although the amount of SAA contained in HDL was not determined in this study [103]. Conflicting with this data others have suggested that SAA does play a role in cholesterol metabolism during acute inflammation [104], although again the relative SAA-to-HDL ratios are not available. It is feasible that SAA can alter HDL function beyond specifically influencing apoA-I concentration, for example by impacting HDL-scavenger receptor VI interactions and scavenger receptor class B member 1 (SR-B1) [71, 105] and / or acting to facilitate the binding

Experimental model	Amount of SAA in HDL	Comments	Ref
Human adipocyte	8-10% SAA in total protein	Slightly induce pro-inflammatory adipose secretion	[102]
ESRD patients	Enriched with SAA, amount not known, apoA-I not detectable.	Reduced anti-inflammatory capacity with reduced MCP-1 inhibition	[92, 93]
C57BL/6 mice	Co-expression of SAA and endothelial lipase	Reduced levels of HDL cholesterol and apo A-I; impeded ABCA1-mediated lipidation of apoA-I	[98]
ACS and CAD subjects	Increased SAA in HDL, amount not known.	Pro-inflammtory profile of HDL in patients; ABCA-1, ABCG-1 and SR-B1 mediated cholesterol efflux are changed	[91]
$SAA^{-/-}$ mice	Amount not available	No impact on HDL cholesterol and apoA-I level	
Human endotoxemia	Unchanged HDL proteome; higher expression of SAA in low HDL-c subjects	Low HDL-c levels are more responsive to inflammatory stimuli compared to high HDL-c	[106]
Mouse HDL	3 apoA-I and 3-5 SAA molecules per HDL particle	Increased binding of HDL to vascular proteoglycans	[71]
U937, THP-1, PBMC, EA.hy. 926 / HuH-7 cells	10-20% SAA in HDL	Increased HDL binding capacity to PBMC / EC	[95]
$SAA^{-/-}$ mice	no SAA level available in HDL	No impact on HDL cholesterol and apoA-I level	[101]
Transgenic mice from C57BL/6	Levels of SAA in HDL not available	No alteration to HDL cholesterol and apoA-I level	[6]
Human THP-1 cells	>50% SAA constituted in HDL	Reduced cellular cholesterol efflux	[17]
$ApoAI^{-/-}$ mice	Overexpression of SAA, only 4% is associated with HDL	Not able to replace apoA-I	[100]

Table 1. Levels of SAA associated in HDL and the influence on HDL activity

of HDL to vascular proteoglycans [71]. Also, SR-B1 mediating is co-expressed with SAA in EC in RA synovial membrane [105] suggesting multiple factors participate in SAA-mediated changes to HDL function.

Independent of the conflicting data on the potential for SAA to impact HDL activity, the relative ratio of SAA to HDL consistently impacts on HDL activity. For example, SAA-induced TNF-α and IL-1β release in THP-1 cells are dose dependently inhibited by the addition of HDL, suggesting that HDL protects against the effects of SAA during SAA transport in the bloodstream [107]. That is, HDL retains its ability to protect HCAEC from SAA stimulation when cells are pre-treated with HDL before addition of pathological SAA [44]. Similarly, endothelium-dependent relaxation was partially restored by pretreatment of aorta with PEG-SOD compared to control (Fig. 4A). Whereas pretreatment of aorta with 100, 200, and 400 (but not 50) μg HDL/mL before stimulation with 10 μg SAA/mL protected from EC dysfunction either partially (~50%) or completely (effective HDL doses *vs* SAA alone; $P < 0.05$, Fig. 4B). Furthermore, reduced NO production in HCAEC stimulated SAA then ACh is restored by pre-incubation of HCAEC with 200 μg HDL/mL before SAA stimulation (see Fig. 2). Conversely, lower HDL-to-SAA ratios are less able to inhibit SAA activity on EC and therefore, increase the likelihood of endothelial dysfunction. The data underscore HDL's protective roles in regulating SAA-mediated damage to EC particularly when high levels of HDL are present relative to SAA.

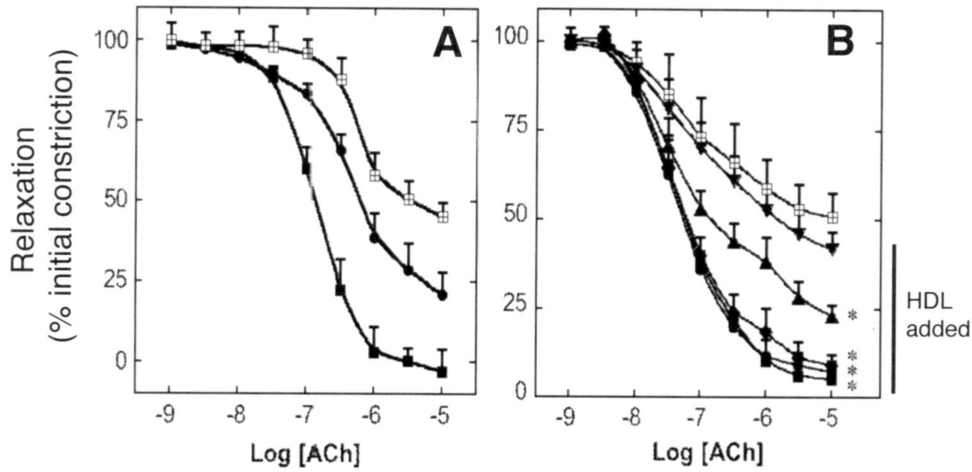

Figure 4. Added PEG-SOD or HDL reverses SAA-provoked vascular dysfunction. Aortic rings were pre-incubated with (A) PEG-SOD (500 U/mL, filled circle) or (B) HDL at 400 (circles), 200 (diamonds), 100 (triangles), or 50 μg/mL (inverted triangles), or vehicle (control). Next, ring segments were treated with vehicle (filled square) or 10 μg SAA/mL (hatched squares) and incubated at 37 °C. After 4 h, rings were treated with phenylephrine and then ACh. Data represent means ± SD, n=5. * P<0.05, different to vessels treated with 10 μg SAA/mL in the absence of HDL.

7. Other actions of SAA on the vascular endothelium

Angiogenesis is defined as the formation of new capillaries from existing vessels, whereas vasculogenesis is a process that involves neo-capillary formation and involves endothelial precursor cells such as angioblast [108]. In addition to activating the vascular endothelium toward pro-inflammatory and pro-thrombotic states, SAA also promotes EC migration and proliferation and this has been linked to its chemokine-like properties that regulate cellular migration and stimulate cell proliferation [69]. The ability of SAA mediating pro-inflammatory response is also to promote neo-capillary formation through a process termed inflammatory angiogenesis [109].

The proliferation of EC is a pathological hallmark of RA where significantly elevated levels of serum SAA and CRP are also a characteristic feature of this pathology [110]. Mullan and co-workers have demonstrated that SAA (i) enhances levels of ICAM-1 and VCAM-1 in RA fibroblast-like synoviocytes (FLS) and human microvascular endothelial cells (HMVECs) and (ii) SAA significantly induces EC tube formation and HMVEC migration emphasising SAA's role in angiogenesis [111]. Presently it is understood that SAA binding to the formyl peptide receptor-like 1 (FPR-1) stimulates this mode of EC activation [112]. Interestingly, activation of FPR-1 by synthetic agonists readily induces macrophage TNF-α production [113] with a parallel increase in ROS production [48]. The latter increases Nfκβ activation [114], which itself enhances TNF-α production [115, 116] and the downstream production of vascular EC growth factor (VEGF) [117]. Furthermore, VEGF signaling activates the expression of EC-derived MMPs that is essential for initiation of EC sprouting [118]. At this point, Notch signaling, an evolutionary conserved protein pathway directing cell-fate determination [119], acts downstream of VEGF signaling to regulate EC morphogenesis via induction and activation of specific MMPs demonstrating that Notch mediates VEGF-induced MMP expression [120]. Notch is also reported to promote extracellular matrix components, such as type I collagen; at the same setting, Notch also induces differentiation of resting fibroblasts into myofibroblasts [121]. In fact, due to high expression Notch 1,2 and 3 in RA patients [122], as well we its particular regulation on cell proliferation and differentiation, Notch is being considered as the direction of a new therapeutic target for RA [123].

Another important mediator: serum amyloid A activating factor-1 (SAF-1), is identified as a critical regulator of a variety of cellular genes including MMP-1 and FLS, and acting as VEGF promoter [124]. Recent studies on experimentally induced arthritis in a SAF-1 transgenic mouse showed a phenotype with markedly higher levels of angiogenesis, synovial inflammation and inflammatory cell infiltration all mediated by induction of VEGF by SAF-1 [125]. SAA-stimulation of ROS production in the endothelium also represents a feasible mechanism that leads to the production of pro-angiogenic factors. Alternately, blockade of SAA binding or direct inhibition to cell surface receptors that binding VEGF may lead to some benefit in this inflammatory condition.

In addition to SAA's participation in angiogenesis during RA, SAA may also be related to the pathogenesis of cancer. Indeed, high levels of SAA in serum concentrations have been associated with gastric [126], lung [127], renal [128] colorectal [129], breast [130], prostatatic [131] and pancreatic cancers [132], where cancer cells themselves have been implicated in localized SAA production. Irrespective of the source of SAA, within the tumor microenvironment, SAA is enriched together with tumor promoting-cytokines produced by activated innate immune cells. Therefore, cancers are likely to stimulate angiogenesis through multiple mechanisms and this should be taken into account in the development of therapeutic drugs that target the inhibition of angiogenesis as a means to limit cancer growth.

8. Future perspectives

Overall, SAA is now increasingly seen as an independent pathogenic risk factor that plays a role in EC activation, and ultimately the development of vascular complications associated with atherosclerosis. Through a concerted relationship with HDL, SAA's pro-atherogenic action on the vascular endothelium may be regulated and this has potential implications for the management of CVD patients that typically show a high SAA/HDL ratio. In terms of clinical impact it is of importance to fully understand the relatioship between native HDL, SAA associated HDL and free SAA and their impact on atherogenesis. Thus, SAA may not be simply a biomarker of inflammatory status, but be actively involved in pro-atherogenic activation of the vascular endothelium.

http://dx.doi.org/10.5772/56047

Abbreviations

ABCG1, ATP-binding cassette sub-family G member 1; ACh, Acetylcholine; ACS, Acute coronary syndrome; apoA-I, Apolipoprotein A-I; apoE$^{-/-}$, Apolipoprotein E-deficient; cGMP, Cyclic guanosine monophosphate; CRP, C-reactive protein; CAD, Coronary artery disease; CVD, Cardiovascular disease; DPI, Diphenyliodonium; EC, Endothelial cells; eNOS, Endothelial nitric oxide synthase; ERK1/2, Extracellular-signal-regulated kinases; ESRD, End-stage renal disease; GM-CSF, Granulocyte-macrophage colony-stimulating factor; HCAEC, Human coronary artery endothelial cells; HDL, High-density lipoproteins; ICAM-1, Intracellular adhesion molecule-1; IL, Interleukins; JNK, c-Jun N-terminal kinases; LDL, Low-density lipoproteins; LPS, Lipolysaccaride; MAPK, Mitogen-activated protein kinase; MCP-1, Monocyte chemotactic protein 1; MIP-1α, Macrophage inflammatory protein 1 α; MMP, Matrix metalloproteases; NADPH, Nicotinamide adenine dinucleotide phosphate; NFκB, Nuclear factor kappa beta; NO, Nitric oxide; $O_2^{\bullet -}$, Superoxide radical anion; ODQ, 1*H*-[1,2,4]oxadiazolo-[4,3-*a*]quinoxalin-1-one; PBMC, Peripheral blood mononuclear cells; PEG-SOD, Polyethylene glycol–superoxide dismutase; RA, Rheumatoid arthritis; ROS, Reactive oxygen species; SAA, Serum amyloid A; SNP, s-nitrosopenicillamine; SOD, Superoxide dismutase; SR-B1, Scavenger receptor class B member 1; TF, Tissue factor; TNF, Tumor necrosis factor-α; THP-1, Human acute monocytic leukemia cell line; VCAM-1, Vascular cell adhesion molecule-1; VEGF, Vascular endothelial cell growth factor.

Acknowledgements

This work was funded in part by a National Heart Foundation of Australia grant-in-aid (G11S5787 awarded to PKW and SBF).

Author details

Xiaosuo Wang[1], Xiaoping Cai[1], Saul Benedict Freedman[2] and Paul K. Witting[1*]

*Address all correspondence to: paul.witting@sydney.edu.au

1 Discipline of Pathology, Sydney Medical School, The University of Sydney, NSW, Australia

2 Department of Cardiology, Concord Hospital, Sydney Medical School, University of Sydney, NSW, Australia

References

[1] Steel, D. M, Sellar, G. C, Uhlar, C. M, Simon, S, Debeer, F. C, & Whitehead, A. S. A Constitutively Expressed Serum Amyloid A Protein Gene (SAA4) Is Closely Linked to, and Shares Structural Similarities with, an Acute-Phase Serum Amyloid A Protein Gene (SAA2). Genomics (1993). , 16(2), 447-454.

[2] Meek, R. L, Eriksen, N, & Benditt, E. P. Serum amyloid A in the mouse. Sites of uptake and mRNA expression. Am J Pathol (1989). , 135(2), 411-9.

[3] Jensen, L. E, & Whitehead, A. S. Regulation of serum amyloid A protein expression during the acute-phase response. Biochem J (1998). Pt 3) 489-503.

[4] Hua, S, Song, C, Geczy, C. L, Freedman, S. B, & Witting, P. K. A role for acute-phase serum amyloid A and high-density lipoprotein in oxidative stress, endothelial dysfunction and atherosclerosis. Redox Rep (2009). , 14(5), 187-96.

[5] Kumon, Y, Hosokawa, T, Suehiro, T, Ikeda, Y, Sipe, J. D, & Hashimoto, K. Acute-phase, but not constitutive serum amyloid A (SAA) is chemotactic for cultured human aortic smooth muscle cells. Amyloid (2002). , 9(4), 237-41.

[6] Kindy, M. S, De Beer, M. C, Yu, J, & De Beer, F. C. Expression of Mouse Acute-Phase (SAA1.1) and Constitutive (SAA4) Serum Amyloid A Isotypes : Influence on Lipoprotein Profiles. Arteriosclerosis, Thrombosis, and Vascular Biology (2000). , 20(6), 1543-1550.

[7] Larson, M. A, Wei, S. H, Weber, A, Weber, A. T, & Mcdonald, T. L. Induction of human mammary-associated serum amyloid A3 expression by prolactin or lipopolysaccharide. Biochemical and Biophysical Research Communications (2003). , 301(4), 1030-1037.

[8] Fasshauer, M, Klein, J, Kralisch, S, Klier, M, Lossner, U, Bluher, M, & Paschke, R. Serum amyloid A3 expression is stimulated by dexamethasone and interleukin-6 in 3T3-L1 adipocytes. Journal of Endocrinology (2004). , 183(3), 561-567.

[9] Gabay, C, & Kushner, I. Acute-Phase Proteins and Other Systemic Responses to Inflammation. New England Journal of Medicine (1999). , 340(6), 448-454.

[10] Uhlar, C. M, & Whitehead, A. S. Serum amyloid A, the major vertebrate acute-phase reactant. Eur J Biochem (1999). , 265(2), 501-23.

[11] Lachmann, H. J, Goodman, H. J. B, Gilbertson, J. A, Gallimore, J. R, Sabin, C. A, Gillmore, J. D, & Hawkins, P. N. Natural History and Outcome in Systemic AA Amyloidosis. New England Journal of Medicine (2007). , 356(23), 2361-2371.

[12] King, V. L, Thompson, J, & Tannock, L. R. Serum amyloid A in atherosclerosis. Current Opinion in Lipidology (2011). MOL.0b013e3283488c39., 22(4), 302-307.

[13] Dong, Z, Wu, T, Qin, W, An, C, Wang, Z, Zhang, M, Zhang, Y, Zhang, C, & An, F. Serum amyloid a directly accelerates the progression of atherosclerosis in apolipoprotein e-deficient mice. Mol Med (2011).

[14] Malle, E, Sodin-semrl, S, & Kovacevic, A. Serum amyloid A: an acute-phase protein involved in tumour pathogenesis. Cell Mol Life Sci (2009). , 66(1), 9-26.

[15] Yamada, T, Kakihara, T, Kamishima, T, Fukuda, T, & Kawai, T. Both acute phase and constitutive serum amyloid A are present in atherosclerotic lesions. Pathology International (1996). , 46(10), 797-800.

[16] Chait, A, Han, C. Y, Oram, J. F, & Heinecke, J. W. Thematic review series: The Immune System and Atherogenesis. Lipoprotein-associated inflammatory proteins: markers or mediators of cardiovascular disease? Journal of Lipid Research (2005). , 46(3), 389-403.

[17] Banka, C. L, Yuan, T, De Beer, M. C, Kindy, M, Curtiss, L. K, & De Beer, F. C. Serum amyloid A (SAA): influence on HDL-mediated cellular cholesterol efflux. J Lipid Res (1995). , 36(5), 1058-65.

[18] Filep, J. G, & El Kebir, D. Serum amyloid A as a marker and mediator of acute coronary syndromes. Future Cardiology (2008). , 4(5), 495-504.

[19] Cai, H, Song, C, Endoh, I, Goyette, J, Jessup, W, Freedman, S. B, Mcneil, H. P, & Geczy, C. L. Serum amyloid A induces monocyte tissue factor. J Immunol (2007). , 178(3), 1852-60.

[20] Song, C, Hsu, K, Yamen, E, Yan, W, Fock, J, Witting, P. K, Geczy, C. L, & Freedman, S. B. Serum amyloid A induction of cytokines in monocytes/macrophages and lymphocytes. Atherosclerosis (2009). , 207(2), 374-383.

[21] Song, C, Shen, Y, Yamen, E, Hsu, K, Yan, W, Witting, P. K, Geczy, C. L, & Freedman, S. B. Serum amyloid A may potentiate prothrombotic and proinflammatory events in acute coronary syndromes. Atherosclerosis (2009). , 202(2), 596-604.

[22] Furlaneto, C. J, & Campa, A. A Novel Function of Serum Amyloid A: A Potent Stimulus for the Release of Tumor Necrosis Factor-α, Interleukin-1β, and Interleukin-8 by Human Blood Neutrophil. Biochemical and Biophysical Research Communications (2000). , 268(2), 405-408.

[23] Cassatella, M. A. The production of cytokines by polymorphonuclear neutrophils. Immunology Today (1995). , 16(1), 21-26.

[24] Furie, B, & Furie, B. C. Mechanisms of Thrombus Formation. New England Journal of Medicine (2008). , 359(9), 938-949.

[25] Zhao, Y, Zhou, S, & Heng, C. K. Impact of Serum Amyloid A on Tissue Factor and Tissue Factor Pathway Inhibitor Expression and Activity in Endothelial Cells. Arteriosclerosis, Thrombosis, and Vascular Biology (2007). , 27(7), 1645-1650.

[26] Jijon, H. B, Madsen, K. L, Walker, J. W, Allard, B, & Jobin, C. Serum amyloid A activates NF-κB and proinflammatory gene expression in human and murine intestinal epithelial cells. European Journal of Immunology (2005). , 35(3), 718-726.

[27] Baranova, I. N, Bocharov, A. V, Vishnyakova, T. G, Kurlander, R, Chen, Z, Fu, D, Arias, I. M, Csako, G, Patterson, A. P, Eggerman, T. L, & Is, C. D. a Novel Serum Amyloid A (SAA) Receptor Mediating SAA Binding and SAA-induced Signaling in Human and Rodent Cells. Journal of Biological Chemistry (2010). , 285(11), 8492-8506.

[28] Utoguchi, N, Ikeda, K, Saeki, K, Oka, N, Mizuguchi, H, Kubo, K, Nakagawa, S, & Mayumi, T. Ascorbic acid stimulates barrier function of cultured endothelial cell monolayer. J Cell Physiol (1995). , 163(2), 393-9.

[29] Napoli, C, & Ignarro, L. J. Nitric Oxide and Atherosclerosis. Nitric Oxide (2001). , 5(2), 88-97.

[30] Phinikaridou, A, Andia, M. E, Protti, A, Indermuehle, A, Shah, A, Smith, A, Warley, A, & Botnar, R. M. Noninvasive MRI Evaluation of Endothelial Permeability in Murine Atherosclerosis Using an Albumin-Binding Contrast Agent. Circulation (2012).

[31] Gonzalez, M. A, & Selwyn, A. P. Endothelial function, inflammation, and prognosis in cardiovascular disease. The American Journal of Medicine (2003). Supplement 1): 99-106.

[32] Murdaca, G, Colombo, B. M, Cagnati, P, Gulli, R, Spanò, F, & Puppo, F. Endothelial dysfunction in rheumatic autoimmune diseases. Atherosclerosis (2012).

[33] Ludmer, P. L, Selwyn, A. P, Shook, T. L, Wayne, R. R, Mudge, G. H, Alexander, R. W, & Ganz, P. Paradoxical Vasoconstriction Induced by Acetylcholine in Atherosclerotic Coronary Arteries. New England Journal of Medicine (1986). , 315(17), 1046-1051.

[34] Thomas, S. R, Witting, P. K, & Drummond, G. R. Redox Control of Endothelial Function and Dysfunction: Molecular Mechanisms and Therapeutic Opportunities Antioxidants & Redox Signaling (2008). , 10(10), 1713-1765.

[35] Bredt, D. S. Endogenous nitric oxide synthesis: Biological functions and pathophysiology. Free Radical Research (1999). , 31(6), 577-596.

[36] Ignarro, L. J, Cirino, G, Casini, A, & Napoli, C. Nitric Oxide as a Signaling Molecule in the Vascular System: An Overview. Journal of Cardiovascular Pharmacology (1999). , 34(6), 879-886.

[37] Anderson, T. J, Gerhard, M. D, Meredith, I. T, Charbonneau, F, Delagrange, D, Creager, M. A, Selwyn, A. P, & Ganz, P. Systemic nature of endothelial dysfunction in atherosclerosis. The American journal of cardiology (1995). Supplement 1): 71B-74B.

[38] Stocker, R, & Keaney, J. F. Role of Oxidative Modifications in Atherosclerosis. Physiological Reviews (2004). , 84(4), 1381-1478.

[39] Maron, B. A, Zhang, Y, White, Y, Chan, K, Handy, S. Y, Mahoney, D. E, Loscalzo, C. E, & Leopold, J. J.A. Aldosterone Inactivates the Endothelin-B Receptor via a Cysteinyl Thiol Redox Switch to Decrease Pulmonary Endothelial Nitric Oxide Levels and Modulate Pulmonary Arterial Hypertension. Circulation (2012).

[40] Van Bussel, B. C. T, Soedamah-muthu, S. S, Henry, R. M. A, Schalkwijk, C. G, Ferreira, I, Chaturvedi, N, Toeller, M, Fuller, J. H, & Stehouwer, C. D. A. Unhealthy dietary patterns associated with inflammation and endothelial dysfunction in type 1 diabetes: The EURODIAB study. Nutrition, Metabolism and Cardiovascular Diseases (2012).

[41] Olsson, N, Siegbahn, A, & Nilsson, G. Serum Amyloid A Induces Chemotaxis of Human Mast Cells by Activating a Pertussis Toxin-Sensitive Signal Transduction Pathway. Biochemical and Biophysical Research Communications (1999). , 254(1), 143-146.

[42] Badolato, R, Johnston, J. A, Wang, J. M, Mcvicar, D, Xu, L. L, Oppenheim, J. J, & Kelvin, D. J. Serum amyloid A induces calcium mobilization and chemotaxis of human monocytes by activating a pertussis toxin-sensitive signaling pathway. The Journal of Immunology (1995). , 155(8), 4004-10.

[43] Lakota, K, Resnik, N, Mrak-poljsak, K, Sodin-semrl, S, & Veranic, P. Colocalization of serum amyloid a with microtubules in human coronary artery endothelial cells. J Biomed Biotechnol (2011).

[44] Witting, P. K, Song, C, Hsu, K, Hua, S, Parry, S. N, Aran, R, Geczy, C, & Freedman, S. B. The acute-phase protein serum amyloid A induces endothelial dysfunction that is inhibited by high-density lipoprotein. Free Radic Biol Med (2011). , 51(7), 1390-8.

[45] Wang, X, Chai, H, Wang, Z, Lin, P. H, Yao, Q, & Chen, C. Serum amyloid A induces endothelial dysfunction in porcine coronary arteries and human coronary artery endothelial cells. Am J Physiol Heart Circ Physiol (2008). H, 2399-408.

[46] Zhao, Y, & Brandish, P. E. DiValentin, M., Schelvis, J.P.M., Babcock, G.T., and Marletta, M.A. Inhibition of Soluble Guanylate Cyclase by ODQ†. Biochemistry (2000). , 39(35), 10848-10854.

[47] Witting, P. K, Rayner, B. S, Wu, B. J, Ellis, N. A, & Stocker, R. Hydrogen Peroxide Promotes Endothelial Dysfunction by Stimulating Multiple Sources of Superoxide Anion Radical Production and Decreasing Nitric Oxide Bioavailability. Cellular Physiology and Biochemistry (2007). , 20(5), 255-268.

[48] Björkman, L, Karlsson, J, Karlsson, A, Rabiet, M, Boulay, J, Fu, F, Bylund, H, & Dahlgren, J. C. Serum amyloid A mediates human neutrophil production of reactive oxygen species through a receptor independent of formyl peptide receptor like-1. Journal of Leukocyte Biology (2008). , 83(2), 245-253.

[49] Cathcart, M. K. Regulation of Superoxide Anion Production by NADPH Oxidase in Monocytes/Macrophages. Arteriosclerosis, Thrombosis, and Vascular Biology (2004). , 24(1), 23-28.

[50] Thomas, S. R, Witting, P. K, & Drummond, G. R. Redox control of endothelial function and dysfunction: molecular mechanisms and therapeutic opportunities. Antioxid Redox Signal (2008). , 10(10), 1713-65.

[51] Brennan, L. A, Steinhorn, R. H, Wedgwood, S, Mata-greenwood, E, Roark, E. A, Russell, J. A, & Black, S. M. Increased Superoxide Generation Is Associated With Pulmonary Hypertension in Fetal Lambs. Circulation Research (2003). , 92(6), 683-691.

[52] Jin, N, & Rhoades, R. A. Activation of tyrosine kinases in H2Oinduced contraction in pulmonary artery. Am J Physiol (1997). Pt 2): H2686-92., 2.

[53] Ülker, S, Mcmaster, D, Mckeown, P. P, & Bayraktutan, U. Impaired activities of antioxidant enzymes elicit endothelial dysfunction in spontaneous hypertensive rats despite enhanced vascular nitric oxide generation. Cardiovascular Research (2003). , 59(2), 488-500.

[54] Griendling, K. K, & Ushio-fukai, M. NADH/NADPH Oxidase and Vascular Function. Trends in Cardiovascular Medicine (1997). , 7(8), 301-307.

[55] Pieper, G. M, Langenstroer, P, & Siebeneich, W. Diabetic-induced endothelial dysfunction in rat aorta: role of hydroxyl radicals. Cardiovascular Research (1997). , 34(1), 145-156.

[56] Wassmann, S, Wassmann, K, & Nickenig, G. Modulation of Oxidant and Antioxidant Enzyme Expression and Function in Vascular Cells. Hypertension (2004). , 44(4), 381-386.

[57] Ohashi, M, Runge, M. S, Faraci, F. M, & Heistad, D. D. MnSOD Deficiency Increases Endothelial Dysfunction in ApoE-Deficient Mice. Arteriosclerosis, Thrombosis, and Vascular Biology (2006). , 26(10), 2331-2336.

[58] Huang, A, Yang, Y, Yan, M, Kaley, C, Hintze, G, & Sun, T. H. D. Altered MAPK Signaling in Progressive Deterioration of Endothelial Function in Diabetic Mice. Diabetes (2012). , 61(12), 3181-3188.

[59] Shatanawi, A, Romero, M. J, Iddings, J. A, Chandra, S, Umapathy, N. S, Verin, A. D, Caldwell, R. B, & Caldwell, R. W. Angiotensin II-induced vascular endothelial dysfunction through RhoA/Rho kinase/mitogen-activated protein kinase/arginase pathway. American Journal of Physiology- Cell Physiology (2011). C1181-C1192., 38.

[60] Schulz, E, Anter, E, & Keaney, J. F. Jr. Oxidative stress, antioxidants, and endothelial function. Curr Med Chem (2004). , 11(9), 1093-104.

[61] Zhang, C, Wu, J, Xu, X, Potter, B. J, & Gao, X. Direct relationship between levels of TNF-alpha expression and endothelial dysfunction in reperfusion injury. Basic Res Cardiol (2010). , 105(4), 453-64.

[62] Jousilahti, P, Salomaa, V, Rasi, V, Vahtera, E, & Palosuo, T. The association of c-reactive protein, serum amyloid a and fibrinogen with prevalent coronary heart disease-baseline findings of the PAIS project. Atherosclerosis (2001). , 156(2), 451-456.

[63] Ridker, P. M, Hennekens, C. H, & Buring, J. E. and Rifai, N. C-Reactive Protein and Other Markers of Inflammation in the Prediction of Cardiovascular Disease in Women. New England Journal of Medicine (2000). , 342(12), 836-843.

[64] Erren, M, Reinecke, H, Junker, R, Fobker, M, Schulte, H, Schurek, J. O, Kropf, J, Kerber, S, Breithardt, G, Assmann, G, & Cullen, P. Systemic Inflammatory Parameters in Patients With Atherosclerosis of the Coronary and Peripheral Arteries. Arteriosclerosis, Thrombosis, and Vascular Biology (1999). , 19(10), 2355-2363.

[65] Johnson, B. D, Kip, K. E. Marroquin, O. C, Ridker, P. M, Kelsey, S. F, Shaw, L. J, Pepine, C. J, & Sharaf, B. Bairey Merz, C.N., Sopko, G., Olson, M.B., and Reis, S.E. Serum Amyloid A as a Predictor of Coronary Artery Disease and Cardiovascular Outcome in Women. Circulation (2004). , 109(6), 726-732.

[66] Leinonen, E, Hurt-camejo, E, Wiklund, O, Hultén, L. M, Hiukka, A, & Taskinen, M. R. Insulin resistance and adiposity correlate with acute-phase reaction and soluble cell adhesion molecules in type 2 diabetes. Atherosclerosis (2003). , 166(2), 387-394.

[67] Haffner, S. M. Agostino Jr, R.D., Saad, M.F., O'Leary, D.H., Savage, P.J., Rewers, M., Selby, J., Bergman, R.N., and Mykkänen, L. Carotid artery atherosclerosis in type-2 diabetic and nondiabetic subjects with and without symptomatic coronary artery disease (The Insulin Resistance Atherosclerosis Study). The American journal of cardiology (2000). , 85(12), 1395-1400.

[68] Connolly, M, Veale, D. J, & Fearon, U. Acute serum amyloid A regulates cytoskeletal rearrangement, cell matrix interactions and promotes cell migration in rheumatoid arthritis. Annals of the Rheumatic Diseases (2011). , 70(7), 1296-1303.

[69] Connolly, M, Marrelli, A, Blades, M, Mccormick, J, Maderna, P, Godson, C, & Mullan, R. FitzGerald, O., Bresnihan, B., Pitzalis, C., Veale, D.J., and Fearon, U. Acute serum amyloid A induces migration, angiogenesis, and inflammation in synovial cells in vitro and in a human rheumatoid arthritis/SCID mouse chimera model. J Immunol (2010). , 184(11), 6427-37.

[70] Lewis, G. F, & Rader, D. J. New Insights Into the Regulation of HDL Metabolism and Reverse Cholesterol Transport. Circulation Research (2005). , 96(12), 1221-1232.

[71] Chiba, T, Chang, M. Y, Wang, S, Wight, T. N, Mcmillen, T. S, Oram, J. F, Vaisar, T, Heinecke, J. W, De Beer, F. C, De Beer, M. C, & Chait, A. Serum Amyloid A Facilitates the Binding of High-Density Lipoprotein From Mice Injected With Lipopolysac-

charide to Vascular Proteoglycans. Arteriosclerosis, Thrombosis, and Vascular Biology (2011). , 31(6), 1326-1332.

[72] Ancsin, J. B, & Kisilevsky, R. The Heparin/Heparan Sulfate-binding Site on Apo-serum Amyloid A. Journal of Biological Chemistry (1999). , 274(11), 7172-7181.

[73] Steinberg, D, Parthasarathy, S, Carew, T. E, Khoo, J. C, & Witztum, J. L. Beyond Cholesterol. New England Journal of Medicine (1989). , 320(14), 915-924.

[74] Wang, X. S, Shao, B, Oda, M. N, Heinecke, J. W, Mahler, S, & Stocker, R. A sensitive and specific ELISA detects methionine sulfoxide-containing apolipoprotein A-I in HDL. Journal of Lipid Research (2009). , 50(3), 586-594.

[75] Coetzee, G. A, Strachan, A. F, Van Der Westhuyzen, D. R, Hoppe, H. C, Jeenah, M. S, & De Beer, F. C. Serum amyloid A-containing human high density lipoprotein 3. Density, size, and apolipoprotein composition. Journal of Biological Chemistry (1986). , 261(21), 9644-9651.

[76] Whitehead, A. S, De Beer, M. C, Steel, D. M, Rits, M, Lelias, J. M, Lane, W. S, & De Beer, F. C. Identification of novel members of the serum amyloid A protein superfamily as constitutive apolipoproteins of high density lipoprotein. Journal of Biological Chemistry (1992). , 267(6), 3862-3867.

[77] Van Lenten, B. J, Wagner, A. C, Navab, M, Anantharamaiah, G. M, Hama, S, Reddy, S. T, & Fogelman, A. M. Lipoprotein inflammatory properties and serum amyloid A levels but not cholesterol levels predict lesion area in cholesterol-fed rabbits. Journal of Lipid Research (2007). , 48(11), 2344-2353.

[78] Yamamoto, K, Shiroo, M, & Migita, S. Diverse gene expression for isotypes of murine serum amyloid A protein during acute phase reaction. Science (1986). , 232(4747), 227-9.

[79] Mucchiano, G. I, Jonasson, L, Häggqvist, B, Einarsson, E, & Westermark, P. Apolipoprotein A-I-Derived Amyloid in Atherosclerosis. American Journal of Clinical Pathology (2001). , 115(2), 298-303.

[80] Lewis, K. E, Kirk, E. A, Mcdonald, T. O, Wang, S, Wight, T. N, Brien, O, & Chait, K. D. A. Increase in Serum Amyloid A Evoked by Dietary Cholesterol Is Associated With Increased Atherosclerosis in Mice. Circulation (2004). , 110(5), 540-545.

[81] Plump, A. S, Smith, J. D, Hayek, T, Aalto-setälä, K, Walsh, A, Verstuyft, J. G, Rubin, E. M, & Breslow, J. L. Severe hypercholesterolemia and atherosclerosis in apolipoprotein E-deficient mice created by homologous recombination in ES cells. Cell (1992). , 71(2), 343-353.

[82] Meir, K. S, & Leitersdorf, E. Atherosclerosis in the Apolipoprotein E-Deficient Mouse. Arteriosclerosis, Thrombosis, and Vascular Biology (2004). , 24(6), 1006-1014.

[83] Letters, J. M, Witting, P. K, Christison, J. K, Eriksson, A. W, Pettersson, K, & Stocker, R. Time-dependent changes to lipids and antioxidants in plasma and aortas of apolipoprotein E knockout mice. Journal of Lipid Research (1999). , 40(6), 1104-1112.

[84] King, V. L, Hatch, N. W, Chan, H, De Beer, W, De Beer, M. C, & Tannock, F. C. L.R. A Murine Model of Obesity With Accelerated Atherosclerosis. Obesity (2009). , 18(1), 35-41.

[85] Ko, K. W. S, Corry, D. B, Brayton, C. F, Paul, A, & Chan, L. Extravascular inflammation does not increase atherosclerosis in apoE-deficient mice. Biochemical and Biophysical Research Communications (2009). , 384(1), 93-99.

[86] Daugherty, A. Mouse Models of Atherosclerosis. The American Journal of the Medical Sciences (2002). , 323(1), 3-10.

[87] Khovidhunkit, W, Kim, M, Memon, S, Shigenaga, R. A, Moser, J. K, Feingold, A. H, & Grunfeld, K. R. C. Thematic review series: The Pathogenesis of Atherosclerosis. Effects of infection and inflammation on lipid and lipoprotein metabolism mechanisms and consequences to the host. Journal of Lipid Research (2004). , 45(7), 1169-1196.

[88] Artl, A, Marsche, G, Lestavel, S, Sattler, W, & Malle, E. Role of Serum Amyloid A During Metabolism of Acute-Phase HDL by Macrophages. Arteriosclerosis, Thrombosis, and Vascular Biology (2000). , 20(3), 763-772.

[89] Benditt, E. P, & Eriksen, N. Amyloid protein SAA is associated with high density lipoprotein from human serum. Proc Natl Acad Sci U S A (1977). , 74(9), 4025-8.

[90] Barter, P. J, Nicholls, S, Rye, K, Anantharamaiah, A, Navab, G. M, & Fogelman, M. A.M. Antiinflammatory Properties of HDL. Circulation Research (2004). , 95(8), 764-772.

[91] Alwaili, K, Bailey, D, Awan, Z, Bailey, S. D, Ruel, I, Hafiane, A, Krimbou, L, Laboissiere, S, & Genest, J. The HDL proteome in acute coronary syndromes shifts to an inflammatory profile. Biochimica et Biophysica Acta (BBA)- Molecular and Cell Biology of Lipids (2012). , 1821(3), 405-415.

[92] Tölle, M, Huang, T, Schuchardt, M, Jankowski, V, Prüfer, N, Jankowski, J, Tietge, U. J. F, Zidek, W, & Van Der Giet, M. High-density lipoprotein loses its anti-inflammatory capacity by accumulation of pro-inflammatory-serum amyloid A. Cardiovascular Research (2012). , 94(1), 154-162.

[93] Weichhart, T, Kopecky, C, Kubicek, M, Haidinger, M, Döller, D, Katholnig, K, Suarna, C, Eller, P, Tölle, M, Gerner, C, Zlabinger, G. J, Van Der Giet, M, Hörl, W. H, Stocker, R, & Säemann, M. D. Serum Amyloid A in Uremic HDL Promotes Inflammation. Journal of the American Society of Nephrology (2012). , 23(5), 934-947.

[94] Kisilevsky, R, & Subrahmanyan, L. Serum amyloid A changes high density lipoprotein's cellular affinity. A clue to serum amyloid A's principal function. Lab Invest (1992). , 66(6), 778-85.

[95] Hayat, S, & Raynes, J. G. Acute phase serum amyloid A protein increases high density lipoprotein binding to human peripheral blood mononuclear cells and an endothelial cell line. Scand J Immunol (2000). , 51(2), 141-6.

[96] Duffy, D, & Rader, D. J. Update on strategies to increase HDL quantity and function. Nat Rev Cardiol (2009). , 6(7), 455-463.

[97] Bailey, D, Jahagirdar, R, Gordon, A, Hafiane, A, Campbell, S, Chatur, S, Wagner, G. S, Hansen, H. C, Chiacchia, F. S, Johansson, J, Krimbou, L, Wong, N. C, & Genest, J. RVX-208: a small molecule that increases apolipoprotein A-I and high-density lipoprotein cholesterol in vitro and in vivo. J Am Coll Cardiol (2010). , 55(23), 2580-9.

[98] Wroblewski, J. M, Jahangiri, A, Ji, A, De Beer, F. C, Van Der Westhuyzen, D. R, & Webb, N. R. Nascent HDL formation by hepatocytes is reduced by the concerted action of serum amyloid A and endothelial lipase. Journal of Lipid Research (2011). , 52(12), 2255-2261.

[99] Kisilevsky, R, & Manley, P. N. Acute-phase serum amyloid A: Perspectives on its physiological and pathological roles. Amyloid (2012). , 19(1), 5-14.

[100] Webb, N. R, De Beer, M. C, Van Der Westhuyzen, D. R, Kindy, M. S, Banka, C. L, Tsukamoto, K, Rader, D. L, & De Beer, F. C. Adenoviral vector-mediated overexpression of serum amyloid A in apoA-I-deficient mice. Journal of Lipid Research (1997). , 38(8), 1583-90.

[101] De Beer, M. C, Webb, N. R, Wroblewski, J. M, Noffsinger, V. P, Rateri, D. L, Ji, A, Van Der Westhuyzen, D. R, & De Beer, F. C. Impact of serum amyloid A on high density lipoprotein composition and levels. Journal of Lipid Research (2010). , 51(11), 3117-3125.

[102] Faty, A, Ferre, P, & Commans, S. The acute phase protein Serum Amyloid A induces lipolysis and inflammation in human adipocytes through distinct pathways. PLoS One (2012). e34031.

[103] De Beer, M. C, Ji, A, Jahangiri, A, Vaughan, A. M, De Beer, F. C, Van Der Westhuyzen, D. R, & Webb, N. R. ATP binding cassette G1-dependent cholesterol efflux during inflammation. Journal of Lipid Research (2011). , 52(2), 345-353.

[104] Lindhorst, E, Young, D, Bagshaw, W, Hyland, M, & Kisilevsky, R. Acute inflammation, acute phase serum amyloid A and cholesterol metabolism in the mouse. Biochimica et Biophysica Acta (BBA)- Protein Structure and Molecular Enzymology (1997). , 1339(1), 143-154.

[105] Mullan, R. H, Mccormick, J, Connolly, M, Bresnihan, B, Veale, D. J, & Fearon, U. A Role for the High-Density Lipoprotein Receptor SR-B1 in Synovial Inflammation via Serum Amyloid-A. The American Journal of Pathology (2010). , 176(4), 1999-2008.

[106] Levels, J. H, Geurts, P, Karlsson, H, Maree, R, Ljunggren, S, Fornander, L, Wehenkel, L, Lindahl, M, Stroes, E. S, Kuivenhoven, J. A, & Meijers, J. C. High-density lipoprotein proteome dynamics in human endotoxemia. Proteome Sci (2011).

[107] Franco, A. G, Sandri, S, & Campa, A. High-density lipoprotein prevents SAA-induced production of TNF-± in THP-1 monocytic cells and peripheral blood mononuclear cells. MemÃ³rias do Instituto Oswaldo Cruz (2011). , 106-986.

[108] Patan, S. Vasculogenesis and angiogenesis. Cancer Treat Res (2004). , 117-3.

[109] Szekanecz, Z, Besenyei, T, Szentpétery, Á, & Koch, A. E. Angiogenesis and vasculogenesis in rheumatoid arthritis. Current Opinion in Rheumatology (2010). BOR. 0b013e328337c95a., 22(3). 299-306.

[110] Tak, P. P, & Bresnihan, B. The pathogenesis and prevention of joint damage in rheumatoid arthritis: Advances from synovial biopsy and tissue analysis. Arthritis & Rheumatism (2000). , 43(12), 2619-2633.

[111] Mullan, R.H, Bresnihan, B, Golden-Mason, L, Markham, T, Hara, O, & Fitz, R. ., and Fearon, U. Acute-phase serum amyloid A stimulation of angiogenesis, leukocyte recruitment, and matrix degradation in rheumatoid arthritis through an NF-κB-dependent signal transduction pathway. Arthritis & Rheumatism 2006. 54 (1): 105-114.

[112] Lee, M, Yoo, S, Cho, S. -A, Suh, C. -S, Kim, P. -G, & Ryu, W. -U. S.H. Serum Amyloid A Binding to Formyl Peptide Receptor-Like 1 Induces Synovial Hyperplasia and Angiogenesis. The Journal of Immunology (2006). , 177(8), 5585-5594.

[113] Schepetkin, I. A, Kirpotina, L. N, Tian, J, Khlebnikov, A. I, Ye, R. D, & Quinn, M. T. Identification of Novel Formyl Peptide Receptor-Like 1 Agonists That Induce Macrophage Tumor Necrosis Factor α Production. Molecular Pharmacology (2008). , 74(2), 392-402.

[114] Neuzil, J, Witting, P. K, Kontush, A, & Headrick, J. P. Role of vitamin E in nuclear factor-kB and nitric oxide signalling. Encyclopedia of Vitamin E, ed. V. Preedy and R. Watson. London: CABI Publishing. (2006).

[115] Stone, K. P, Kastin, A. J, & Pan, W. NFκB is an Unexpected Major Mediator of Interleukin-15 Signaling in Cerebral Endothelia. Cellular Physiology and Biochemistry (2011). , 28(1), 115-124.

[116] Li, W, Li, H, Bocking, A. D, & Challis, J. R. G. Tumor Necrosis Factor Stimulates Matrix Metalloproteinase 9 Secretion from Cultured Human Chorionic Trophoblast Cells Through TNF Receptor 1 Signaling to IKBKB-NFKB and MAPK1/3 Pathway. Biology of Reproduction (2010). , 83(3), 481-487.

[117] González-pacheco, F. R, Deudero, J. J. P, Castellanos, M. C, Castilla, M. A, Álvarez-arroyo, M. V, Yagüe, S, & Caramelo, C. Mechanisms of endothelial response to oxidative aggression: protective role of autologous VEGF and induction of VEGFR2 by

H2O2. American Journal of Physiology- Heart and Circulatory Physiology (2006). HH1401., 1395.

[118] Hollborn, M, Stathopoulos, C, Steffen, A, Wiedemann, P, Kohen, L, & Bringmann, A. Positive Feedback Regulation between MMP-9 and VEGF in Human RPE Cells. Investigative Ophthalmology & Visual Science (2007). , 48(9), 4360-4367.

[119] Shawber, C. J, & Kitajewski, J. Notch function in the vasculature: insights from zebrafish, mouse and man. BioEssays (2004). , 26(3), 225-234.

[120] Funahashi, Y, Shawber, C, Sharma, A, Kanamaru, E, Choi, Y, & Kitajewski, J. Notch modulates VEGF action in endothelial cells by inducing Matrix Metalloprotease activity. Vascular Cell (2011).

[121] Warde, N. Connective tissue diseases: Notch signaling: an important player in SSc fibrosis. Nat Rev Rheumatol (2011). , 7(6), 312-312.

[122] Ishii, H, Nakazawa, M, Yoshino, S, Nakamura, I, Nishioka, H, & Nakajima, K. T. Expression of Notch homologues in the synovium of rheumatoid arthritis and osteoarthritis patients. Rheumatology International (2001). , 21(1), 10-14.

[123] Sassi, N, Laadhar, L, Driss, M, Kallel-sellami, M, Sellami, S, & Makni, S. The role of the Notch pathway in healthy and osteoarthritic articular cartilage: from experimental models to ex vivo studies. Arthritis Research & Therapy (2011).

[124] Ray, A, Kuroki, K, Cook, J. L, Bal, B. S, Kenter, K, Aust, G, & Ray, B. K. Induction of matrix metalloproteinase 1 gene expression is regulated by inflammation-responsive transcription factor SAF-1 in osteoarthritis. Arthritis & Rheumatism (2003). , 48(1), 134-145.

[125] Ray, A, Kumar, D, Shakya, A, Brown, C. R, Cook, J. L, & Ray, B. K. Serum amyloid A-activating factor-1 (SAF-1) transgenic mice are prone to develop a severe form of inflammation-induced arthritis. J Immunol (2004). , 173(7), 4684-91.

[126] Chan, D, Chen, C, Chu, C. -J, Chang, H. -C, Yu, W. -K, Chen, J. -C, Wen, Y. -J, Huang, L. -L, Ku, S. -C, & Liu, C. -H. Y.-C.e.a. Evaluation of Serum Amyloid A as a Biomarker for Gastric Cancer. Annals of Surgical Oncology (2007). , 14(1), 84-93.

[127] Benson, M, Eyanson, S, & Fineberg, N. Serum amyloid A in carcinoma of the lung. Cancer (1986). , 57(9), 1783-7.

[128] Kimura, M, Tomita, Y, Imai, T, Saito, T, Katagiri, A, Ohara-mikami, Y, Matsudo, T, & Takahashi, K. Significance of serum amyloid A on the prognosis in patients with renal cell carcinoma. Cancer. (2001). , 92(8), 2072-5.

[129] Glojnaric, I, Casl, M, Šimic, T, & Lukac, D. J. Serum Amyloid A Protein (SAA) in Colorectal Carcinoma. Clinical Chemistry and Laboratory Medicine. (2005). , 39(2), 129-133.

http://dx.doi.org/10.5772/56047

[130] Zhang, G, Sun, X, Lv, H, Yang, X, & Kang, X. Serum amyloid A: A new potential serum marker correlated with the stage of breast cancer. Oncol Lett. (2012). , 3(4), 940-944.

[131] Firpo, M, Gay, D, Granger, S, & Scaife, C. DiSario, J., Boucher, K., and Mulvihill, S. Improved diagnosis of pancreatic adenocarcinoma using haptoglobin and serum amyloid A in a panel screen. World J Surg. (2009). , 33(4), 716-722.

[132] Yokoi, K, Shih, L, Kobayashi, C. N, Koomen, R, Hawke, J, Li, D, Hamilton, D, Tanley, S, Abbruzzese, R, Coombes, J. L, & Fidler, K. R. I, s.J. Serum amyloid A as a tumor marker in sera of nude mice with orthotopic human pancreatic cancer and in plasma of patients with pancreatic cancer. Int J Oncol, (2005). , 27, 1361-1369.

Chapter 5

The Use of Acute Phase Proteins as Biomarkers of Diseases in Cattle and Swine

Csilla Tóthová, Oskar Nagy and Gabriel Kováč

Additional information is available at the end of the chapter

http://dx.doi.org/10.5772/55857

1. Introduction

The acute phase response is a nonspecific and complex reaction of an organism that occurs shortly after any tissue injury. The origin of this response can be attributable to infectious, traumatic, immunologic, neoplastic, or other causes, in order to restore homeostasis, reduce tissue damage, and to remove the cause of disturbances [1]. The acute phase response is characterized by a number of different systemic effects, a range of metabolic activities and alterations in a wide variety of biochemical processes. One of the most important metabolic changes is the strongly increased (or decreased) production and secretion of some plasma proteins from the liver, the acute phase proteins [2]. The acute phase response is a very fast response, developing with increased concentrations of acute phase proteins within a few hours, which remain elevated as long as the inflammatory stimulus persists [3]. For this reason, they represent the ideal tool for the early identification of inflammation or injury, and for monitoring the outcome of disease processes. Unfortunately, acute phase proteins are poorly specific, since they increase in the presence of inflammation independent of the agent responsible, but the increase in their concentrations indicates that „something" is happening in the body, and should lead clinician to investigate the site, type and severity of the inflammation (complete clinico-pathological approach), to identify the pathogen responsible (specific diagnostic methods), and to follow-up the treatment.

Acute phase proteins have been studied widely in human medicine, especially as biomarkers of diseases, inflammatory processes and various infections, to diagnose and monitor the success of diseases in clinical praxis [4,5]. However, they have been relatively under-utilised in the veterinary medicine, and the possible influence of inflammatory conditions on the concentrations of these proteins, and they use as indicators in the monitoring of animal health and detection of diseases in veterinary clinical practice, especially in farm animal medicine is less well documented. For this reason, the main purpose of this article is to provide an integrated overview about the diagnostically valuable acute phase proteins in farm animals, to update the knowledge about their usefulness in the detection and diagnosis of various economically important diseases of ruminants and swine, and present some new knowledge regarding their clinical applicability and methods for determination.

2. The acute phase response

The acute phase response is a complex early-defense system induced by any process that leads to tissue damage, e.g. bacterial and viral infection, inflammation, parasite infestation, trauma, surgery, ischemic necrosis, burns, neoplastic growth [6]. The reactions of the acute phase response are part of the non-specific immune system and thus the first line of defense against invading pathogens, which is responsible for the survival of the host during the critical early stages of the attack. It is designed to hold the infection in check until the adaptive, highly specialized immune response is initiated [7]. The acute phase response is a cascade of host responses with the goal of reestablishing the homeostasis, to remove the cause of disturbance and promote the healing process [8].

The pathogenesis of the acute phase response begins within inflammatory sites, where cells involved in the innate immune response (i.e. macrophages, monocytes) produce and release a vast number of inflammatory mediators, among which the cytokines (such as interleukin-1, interleukin-6 and tumor necrosis factor-α) play very important roles [9]. These cytokines influence organs involved in homeostasis, such as the central nervous system (CNS), the autonomic nervous system and the adrenal gland, to establish a rapid and intense protective or reactive response [10]. Cytokines induce a cascade of events which potentiate the appearance of the main clinical changes charecterized by fever, anorexia or weight loss [11]. In addition, the cytokines activate receptors on different target cells leading to systemic inflammatory reactions, including hormonal or metabolic, and resulting in a number of biochemical changes [12]. These symptoms reflect multiple changes in the homeostatic control of the diseased animals, such as increased production of adrenocorticotrophic hormone and glucocorticoids, activation of the complement cascade and blood coagulation system, decreased serum concentrations of calcium, zinc, iron, vitamin A and α-tocopherol, and changes in the concentrations of some plasma proteins [13]. One of the most important metabolic changes is the strongly increased synthesis of a group of plasma proteins, namely acute phase proteins, by the liver [14].

3. Acute phase proteins

In general, the acute phase proteins are a group of blood proteins that change in concentrations in animals subjected to external or internal challenges, such as infection, inflammation, trauma or stress [1]. Acute phase proteins can be classified according to the magnitude of the increase (positive acute phase proteins) or decrease (negative acute phase proteins) in their serum concentrations during the acute phase response [15]. They are further classified as major, moderate, or minor, depending on their responsibility. Major proteins represent those that increase 10- to 100-fold, moderate proteins increase 2- to 10-fold, and minor proteins are characterized with only a slight increase [16]. Major proteins often are observed to increase markedly within the first 24 – 48 hours after the triggering event and often have a rapid decline due to their very short half-life. Moderate and minor proteins follow in magnitude of response and may both increase more slowly and be more prolonged in duration, depending on the status of the triggering event [17]. Moderate and minor acute phase proteins may be observed more often during chronic inflammatory processes [18]. In these cases, an aberrant continuation of some aspects of the acute phase response may contribute to the underlying tissue damage, which accompanies the disease and also may lead to further complications, for example protein deposition such as reactive amyloidosis [19].

Generally, the main function of acute phase proteins is to defend the host against pathological damage and assist in the restoration of the homeostasis. Some of the acute phase proteins (α_1-antitrypsin, α_2-macroglobulin) have anti-protease activity designed to inhibit proteases released by phagocytes or pathogens to minimize damage to normal tissues [13]. Another acute phase proteins (haptoglobin, serum amyloid A, C-reactive protein) have scavenging activities and bind metabolites released from cellular degradation so they can re-enter host metabolic processes rather than be utilized by pathogen [20]. Others (α_1-acid glycoprotein) are characterized by anti-bacterial activity and by the ability to influence the course of the immune response [21].

Despite the uniform nature of the acute phase response, there are numerous differences in the acute phase characteristics between different animal species [13]. The important concept is that each animal species has its own major acute phase proteins that must be considered the markers of choice for diagnostic purposes. Ruminants are significantly different to other species in their acute phase response, in that haptoglobin (Hp) and serum amyloid A (SAA) are the major acute phase proteins [22]. On the other hand, in pigs, significant increases of C-reactive protein have been detected after an inflammatory stimulus [23].

4. The diagnostic utility of acute phase proteins in the veterinary practice

It is important to recognize that acute phase protein concentrations are elevated in animals with many different diseases, having very poor diagnostic specificity in detecting the cause, so they can not be used as the primary diagnostic test for a particular disease. However, they have very high sensitivity in detecting many conditions that alter the health of the animal and in providing evidence that an animal has subclinical inflammation or infection [16]. It was reported by Kent [24] that acute phase proteins quickly and precisely demonstrate the presence of infectious and inflammatory conditions, but not the cause. A very interesting characteristic of the acute phase proteins is the possibility of detecting subclinical diseases [16]. Petersen et al. [15] stated also that acute phase proteins can detect the presence of subclinical disease which is the cause of reduced growth rate and losses in the production. In the clinical field, acute phase proteins may serve as indicators of prognosis and effect of treatment. The magnitude and duration of the acute phase response reflect the severity of the infection and underlying tissue damage [25]

Practical uses and advantages of acute phase protein assays in small animals have been described and demonstrated in a large number of scientific reports published in a last few years. However, clinical application of acute phase proteins in large animals has not been sufficiently standardized in routine practice. The possible use of acute phase proteins in ruminants and swine has been investigated in various inflammatory and non-inflammatory conditions. However, there are many more areas of enquiry which can be pursued to deepen our knowledge about the acute phase response and also to develop novel applications for the acute phase proteins, e.g. during some less frequently studied diseases of young (diarrhoea, omphalophlebitis) and adult cattle (laminitis, mastitis), as well as not only in acute infections, but also in chronic inflammatory conditions. Moreover, the concentrations of acute phase proteins must be interpreted in the view of many other influences not associated with diseases. The age of evaluated animals, parturition, the transition of pregnancy to lactation are important factors that may affect the concentrations of frequently analyzed biochemical variables, including the concentrations of acute phase proteins. Considering that the evaluation of acute phase proteins would be important diagnostic aid available to clinicians, their usefulness for diagnosis and prognosis of various disorders and diseases in cattle and swine will be discussed, including the influence of some physiologic conditions on their values.

4.1. The effect of age on the concentrations of acute phase proteins

After birth, newborns and young animals go through a period of rapid growth and development, and adapt to life outside the uterus. This transition from foetal to neonatal life and then from newborn to young animal necessitates major physiological adjustments [26]. Young calves must adapt to various environmental factors, including nutrition which changes from a primarily carbohydrate-based energy supply during the foetal period to a high fat and relatively low carbohydrate nutritional energy supply in colostrum and milk, and then from milk to solid diet [27]. The exposure to the new environment and foreign antigens requires the establishment of appropriate defence responses [28]. The neonate is immunocompetent, but the adaptive immune system is immature [29]. Non-specific defence mechanisms, including the reactions of the acute phase response may thus be important for the adaptation to complicated physiological processes during growth and development of calves. Therefore, the concentrations of acute phase proteins may be influenced by the age of evaluated animals. The concentrations measured in young calves thus may differ from the values in adult cattle. Therefore, higher concentrations of acute phase proteins, which in adult cattle may indicate an inflammatory process, in young calves are not necessarily a sign of the activation of the acute phase protein production by some inflammatory stimulus, or a sign of a disease.

Possible factors affecting the concentrations of acute phase proteins after birth include foetal synthesis of acute phase proteins, the stimulation of their production by birth trauma, intake of colostrum containing acute phase proteins or their stimulants, and immaturity of synthesis

http://dx.doi.org/10.5772/55857

Variable		Age of the calves (months)						P
		1	2	3	4	5	6	
Hp (mg/ml)	x	0.068^{A}	0.064	0.056	0.213	0.062	0.021^{A}	< 0.05
	± SD	0.021	0.026	0.024	0.344	0.081	0.018	
SAA (µg/ml)	x	59.12^{a}	53.37	39.71	21.20	10.51^{a}	19.86	< 0.05
	± SD	35.61	21.43	26.65	19.97	10.36	27.42	
Fbg (g/l)	x	2.31	3.14^{a}	2.55	2.87	2.82^{b}	2.17^{a,b}	< 0.01
	± SD	0.76	0.75	0.32	0.57	0.40	0.20	

The same superscripts in rows mean statistical significance of differences in concentrations between the columns: a, b – P < 0.05, A – P < 0.01

P – significance of the differences

Table 1. Age-related changes in the concentrations of evaluated acute phase proteins in clinically healthy calves from the 1st till 6th month of age [34]

capacity of the newborn liver [28]. Introduction to the extrauterine environment, which contains various microbes, could also trigger an inflammatory response. Colostrum contains high amount of inflammatory mediators such as cytokines, which may induce the acute phase response in newborns. Transfer of colostral cytokines to the blood of calves has been reported by Yamanaka et al. [30]. In addition, direct transfer of some acute phase proteins from colostrum to newborns may potentially occur. Schroedl et al. [31] found elevated concentrations of CRP in young calves. They concluded that although CRP in cattle is not a major acute phase protein, bovine colostrum contains high amounts of CRP and its transfer contributes to elevated concentrations in newborn calves. Moreover, high concentrations of mammary-associated SAA in the colostrum of healthy cows were found, which have a primarily protective effect on the gastrointestinal tract of neonates by stimulating mucin production and reducing adherence of pathogens [32]. Immaturity of the neonatal liver to mount an acute phase response to an inflammatory stimulus could affect the concentrations of acute phase proteins in neonatal animals. For example, low Hp concentrations are common in newborn infants, which are related to the immaturity of the liver to produce Hp in a situation where Hp consumption is increased because of haemolysis of foetal erythrocytes [33].

Tóthová et al. [34] evaluated the age-dependent changes in the concentrations of haptoglobin (Hp), serum amyloid A (SAA) and fibrinogen (Fbg) in clinically healthy calves during the first 6 month of life. The most pronounced changes they observed in the concentrations of SAA, with the highest concentrations at the age of 1 month followed by gradually decreasing values to 5th month of life (Table 1). Orro et al. [28] reported also higher mean serum concentrations of SAA shortly after birth, being the highest at the age of 7 days (112.0 mg/l), and decreased after 10 days of age. In contrast, low SAA concentrations have been noted by Alsemgeest et al. [35] in calves sampled within 10 min after parturition. The results obtained by Tóthová et al. [34] showed in calves less pronounced changes in the Hp concentrations during the first three months of life than those observed in the serum SAA concentrations. The concentrations of Hp in the blood serum of calves in the first three months after birth were roughly uniform, and the values were comparable with the concentrations measured in healthy adult cattle. Similar findings were reported by Hyvönen et al. *[36]*. Orro et al. [28] also stated that serum Hp concentrations after birth were more stable compared with serum amyloid A. Slightly higher mean Hp concentration was observed by the abovementioned authors at the age of 3 days, and then (after a small decrease) the serum concentrations of Hp remained relatively stabile. Schroedl et al. [31] described that the concentrations of Hp in newborn calves did not differ between samples obtained at birth, at 1 day of age and at 10 days of age. Studies performed by Knowles et al. [37] showed that the concentrations of fibrinogen in calves increased during the first 2 weeks after birth, although the rise was relatively small, and the concentrations did not exceed the general reference limit used for healthy cattle. Very similar transient and relatively small increases in Fbg concentrations during the first 2 weeks of life in calves have been reported by Gentry et al. [38]. The results presented by Tóthová et al. [34] showed a transient increase in the plasma concentrations of fibrinogen at the age of 2 months, which was followed by a repeated decrease of Fbg concentrations, and the obtained values were similar to those usually measured in healthy adult cattle.

5. Acute phase proteins in cattle

5.1. Haptoglobin

Haptoglobin (Hp) is a glycoprotein composed of 2 α and 2 β subunits. The α subunit has a molecular weight of 16 – 23 kDa and the β subunit 35 – 40 kDa. The subunits combine in the form of a β-α-α-β tetramer chain [39]. In the circulation, Hp is highly polymerized having a molecular weight of approximately 1000 – 2000 kDa, and exists also as polymer associated with albumin [40]. The primary function of Hp is to bind free hemoglobin in the blood. By removing from the circulation any free hemoglobin, which has inherent peroxidase activity, Hp prevents oxidative damage to tissues [41]. The Hp-hemoglobin binding also reduces the availability of the heme residue from bacterial growth and therefore Hp has an indirect antibacterial activity [1]. Many studies have indicated the significance of Hp as a clinically useful parameter for measuring the occurrence and severity of inflammatory responses in cattle with mastitis, pneumonia, enteritis, peritonitis, endocarditis, abscesses, endometritis and other natural or experimental infectious conditions [42].

Assays for serum Hp concentration include spectrophotometric methods and immunoassays. The spectrophotometric assays are based on the ability of Hp to bind hemoglobin (Hb), forming Hp-Hb complexes that either alter the absorbance characteristic for Hb in proportion to the concentration of Hp in a serum sample, or preserve peroxidase activity at an acidic pH, which then can be detected and quantified [43]. In addition, an automated spectrophotometric multispecies assay based on this reactivity has been developed [44]. Nephelometric immunoassays, in which the rate of the precipitation of the antibody-antigen complex is measured, have been validated for the estimation of Hp [45].

5.2. Serum amyloid A

Serum amyloid A (SAA) is a small hydrophobic protein (9 – 14 kDa), which is found in serum associated with high density lipoprotein. In humans, four separate isoforms have been identified [46]. Of these, SAA1 and SAA2 respond to an acute phase reaction with increased production from the liver. In contrast, SAA4 is a constitutive protein that is produced normally at low concentrations and is not affected by the acute phase response. The SAA3 isoform is expressed in non-hepatic tissues during the acute phase response with increases found in lung, adipose tissue, ovarian granulosa, as well as in the mammary gland [47]. The mammary isoform (M-SAA3) has also been detected in bovine colostrum [32]. Among the functions ascribed to SAA have been reverse transport of cholesterol from tissue to hepatocytes, opsonisation, inhibition of phagocyte oxidative burst and platelet activation [15]. The M-SAA3 isoform found in colostrum stimulates the production of mucin from intestinal cells assisting the initiation of secretions from the neonatal intestine and helping to prevent bacterial colonization [48].

Enzyme linked immunosorbent assay (ELISA) is the commonest format for immunoassays of SAA. A cross species SAA immunoassay has been developed for measuring in veterinary medicine, that can be used in most species as the antibody shows species specificity for SAA [49]. In addition, the latex agglutination test and turbidimetric immunoassay has been validated for SAA determination [50].

5.3. Fibrinogen

Fibrinogen (Fbg), a precursor of fibrin, is also an acute phase protein, which has been used for many years to evaluate inflammatory and traumatic diseases in cattle, and is characterized by markedly increased synthesis in response to infection [51]. Fibrinogen is a β-globulin present in the plasma. It is composed of 3 polypeptide chains linked by disulfide bridges and a glycoprotein [52]. Fibrinogen is involved in homeostasis, providing a substrate for fibrin formation, and in tissue repair, providing a matrix for the migration of inflammatory-related cells [53]. Assays for fibrinogen have been largely dependent on its biological activity based on the rate of formation of insoluble fibrin in the presence of excess thrombin or on its precipitation following mild heat treatment [54].

5.4. Albumin

Serum albumin is the major negative acute phase protein. During the acute phase response the demand for amino acids for synthesis of the positive acute phase proteins is markedly increased, which necessitates reprioritization of the hepatic protein synthesis: albumin synthesis is down-regulated and amino acids are shunted into synthesis of positive acute phase proteins [55]. It has been reported that during the acute phase response 30 to 40 % of the hepatic protein synthesizing capacity is used for production of positive acute phase proteins and the production of other proteins thus need to be diminished [56]. Albumin is responsible for about 75 % of the osmotic pressure of plasma and is a major source of amino acids that can be utilized by the animal's body when necessary. In routine practice, albumin is usually measured by spectrophotometric methods, such as the bromcresol green assay. However, overestimation of albumin can occur in heparinized plasma samples assayed by this method [57].

6. Acute phase proteins in pigs

In the pigs, C-reactive protein, haptoglobin, α_1-acid glycoprotein, and pig specific major acute phase protein were identified as the diagnostically most important acute phase proteins.

6.1. C-reactive protein

In the pigs, as in the dogs and humans, C-reactive protein (CRP) is the prototypical acute phase protein with major diagnostic value. This protein was the first acute phase protein to be described. Originally named for its ability to bind the C-polysaccharide of *Streptococcus pneumoniae*, CRP has been defined as an exquisitely sensitive systemic marker of inflammation and tissue damage [58]. C-reactive protein plays important roles in the protection against infection, clearence of damaged tissues, and regulation of the inflammatory response [59]. Structurally, CRP is a cyclic pentamer which binds with a variety of pathogenic bacteria or intracellular antigens of damaged cells, thus recognising foreign molecules and altered self [1].

Measurement of serum CRP is generally by immunoassays using specific CRP antibodies, and several formats have been developed and described for this purpose, such as immunoturbidimetric assay, ELISA, or latex agglutination tests [60,61]. Currently, a commercial ELISA kit is available that is specific for porcine CRP, although technical improvements are needed to decrease between-run imprecision.

6.2. Alpha$_1$-acid glycoprotein

The main biochemical characteristic of α_1-acid glycoprotein (AGP) is that it is a highly glycosylated protein and is the main protein component in seromucoid [62]. It does bind to a number of metabolites such as heparin, histamine and serotonin, steroids and catecholamines [63]. AGP is also known to bind to pharmacological compounds which may have therapeutic implications as the amount bound can affect the metabolically active fraction of the drug. Increased AGP due to an acute phase response thus may reduce the concentration of free drugs, thus affecting their pharmacokinetics.

Although AGP can be estimated by precipitation of the majority of serum proteins by perchloric acid and quantification of the remaining soluble proteins, this protein is usually measured by single radial immunodiffusion on agarose gel impregnated with anti-species AGP rabbit serum [64]. These tests are species-specific; however, they have the disadvantage of requiring 24 or 48 hours for diffusion to be complete.

6.3. Pig specific major acute phase protein

Specifically in the pigs, this specific acute phase protein (pig MAP) of unknown function has been reported to be a sensitive indicator of infection. Increases in pig MAP have been shown during infections with *Actinobacillus pleuropneumoniae*, in post weaning multisystemic wasting disorder and following transport [65]. The application of this protein to the veterinary diagnosis seems promising but needs further investigation.

7. Acute phase proteins in cattle diseases

7.1. Acute phase proteins in calves

7.1.1. Acute phase proteins in calves with respiratory diseases

Respiratory diseases are one of the leading causes of morbidity and mortality in calves and young cattle, and may account for serious economic losses [66]. In case of dairy calf pneumonia, diagnosis and treatment are mainly based on the observation of clinical symptoms, such as depression and body temperature combined with specific disease signs. However, in many cases, the infected calves show only mild clinical symptoms that could be easily missed in a group of calves on a farm [67]. To prevent disease outbreaks, early detection, isolation and treatment of diseased animals is important. Therefore, there is a need for objective parameters that are suitable as indicators of health or disease in calf herds applicable in the laboratory diagnosis of diseases. These proteins have been found to increase in the serum of cattle with many different diseases, including experimentally induced and naturally occurring respiratory tract diseases [40].

Respiratory-tract diseases are considered to be multi-factorial with causative agents, calf factors and environmental factors. The most common agents found in association with respiratory diseases are viruses such as bovine respiratory syncytial virus (BRSV), bovine herpesvirus (BHV-1), parainfluenza- virus (PI-3). On the other hand, secondary bacterial infections, e.g. *Mannheimia haemolytica, Pasteurella multocida, Histophilus somni* are common [68]. However, scientist are not in agreement as to whether bacterial or viral infections mount a higher response. Conner et al. [69] showed that intra-tracheal aerosol inoculation with *Mannheimia (M.) haemolytica* in calves raised the levels of haptoglobin, α_1-antitrypsin, and seromucoid. The aforementioned authors showed the earliest detectable rise in the concentrations of Hp after 24 hours, with the highest value on day 3 after inoculation (1.0 g/l). Similar to previous data reported by Makimura and Suzuki [43], the Hp concentrations were undetectable (less than 30 μg/ml) in animals prior to challenge. These data provide valuable information regarding the induction and kinetics of haptoglobin production. Horadagoda and Eckersall [70] evaluated also calves intra-tracheally infected with *M. haemolytica* serotype A1. The results reported by these authors showed a small, insignificant increase in Hp concentrations within 10 h post-inoculation. In contrast, the concentrations of serum amyloid A increased progressively from undetectable values at inoculation to 18 mg/l measured 10 hours after the infection. These data indicate that SAA is a more rapidly reacting acute phase protein compared to haptoglobin in response to bacterial infection with *M. haemolytica*. On the other hand, Angen et al. [71] reported that even if SAA is more rapidly reacting acute phase protein, it needs virus to be present in order to respond, while Hp is fully induced by bacterial infection alone.

Godson et al. [40] investigated the serum protein profile from animals with bovine respiratory diseases to identify bovine acute phase proteins which may be used as indicators of the disease. For this reason, they experimentally reproduced bovine respiratory diseases, by challenging seronegative calves with bovine herpesvirus (BHV-1) on day 0 and *M. haemolytica* A-1 strain on day 4, which mimics the clinical signs and pathological changes associated with the naturally occuring fibrinous pneumonia observed in feedlots. In this model of virus induced bacterial pneumonia, the aforementioned authors found only few animals responding to the viral challenge with increased haptoglobin concentrations. Over the first 4 days after BHV-1 exposure, only 10 % of animals developed Hp concentrations higher than 100 μg/ml. However, 24 hours after *M. haemolytica* challenge, 43 % of the animals had Hp values in excess of 100 μg/ml, and 3 days after challenge, this proportion reached 84 %. Moreover, the proportion of animals responding and the mean Hp concentration continued to rise for another 2 – 3 days. Thus, according to Godson et al. [40], haptoglobin induction appeared to be related to the onset of bacterial infection. Moreover, in the aforementioned study, the induction of haptoglobin production was temporally associated with the development of the disease, as well as the disease severity (fever, sick score, weight loss). While all animals which were clinically sick had elevated Hp concentrations, increased Hp values were detected also in some animals that did not show apparent illness. Thus, the measurement of Hp may detect infected animals before clinical signs of the disease become apparent [25]. Furthermore, Godson et al. [40] reported significantly higher Hp concentration in animals that subsequently died compared to those that recovered. Similar findings were reported by Tóthová et al. [72] in calves suffering from bovine respiratory disease under field conditions. Therefore, the determination of Hp concentrations may serve as a prognostic aid in determining the severity of the disease. Further examination of the acute phase response of calves to bacterial infection with *Pasteurella multocida* biotype A3 was performed by Dowling et al. [73] to describe the changes in acute phase reactants of the host to either low or high volumes of the inocula. The results of the aforementioned authors showerd that all treatments elicited a moderate to severe response and induced clinical signs characteristic of bovine pneumonic pasteurellosis as observed in natural cases. However, the results of the acute phase reactants indicated that, of the two treatment variables used (dose and volume), volume was the more influential factor inducing the disease. In calves challenged with greater volumes (300 vs. 60 ml) they found significantly higher Hp concentrations, regardless of the number of the bacteria (10^9 vs. 10^{10} cfu). Dowling et al. [73] expected that increased volume challenges affect a greater area of the lungs, especially if the initially slow response in Hp production provides more time for bacterial proliferation. Moreover, they stated that the increases in the concentrations of α_1-acid glycoprotein were more gradual than those observed for Hp and maintained for longer period.

Heegaard et al. [25] evaluated the acute phase response of calves to experimental viral infection with bovine respiratory syncytial virus (BRSV). While the serum concentrations of both serum amyloid A and haptoglobin remained low in all control animals in this study, the SAA concentrations became elevated in the most of experimentally infected animals. This elevation was detectable at day 5 after infection, and peaked around day 5 – 8 *post infection*. The highest SAA concentrations were in the range of 60 – 80 μg/ml, which is about 5 – 7 times higher than the values obtained in the control animals. Generally, changes in Hp concentrations followed the changes in SAA values. The maximum response of Hp was seen on day 6 -7 after infection, and reached 8 – 10 mg/ml. In the study by Heegaard et al. [25], SAA responded more rapidly to infection, but Hp concentrations correlated better with disease severity. Similar findings were reported by Grell et al. [74] in calves experimentally infected with BRSV with the highest Hp concentrations at 7 – 9 days after inoculation. Moreover, calves with the most severe clinical symptoms had the highest Hp values. Gänheim et al. [67] examined the acute phase response in calves experimentally infected in the respiratory tract with either bovine viral diarrhoea virus (BVDV) or *M. haemolytica*, or with a combination of the two agents. They investigated also the differences in the magnitude and kinetics between single and dual infection. In all inoculated groups, a significant acute phase response was observed with elevated values of Hp, SAA, as well as fibrinogen, while the control group remained unaffected throughout the study. In general, the magnitude of the response was similar, but the duration of increased concentrations of measured acute phase proteins were the longest in the BVDV/*M. haemolytica* group, reflecting the duration of the clinical symptoms. According to the data obtained by Gänheim et al. [67], the acute phase response occured much faster after *M. haemolytica* inoculation than after BVDV infection. After BVDV inoculation, increases in the acute phase protein concentrations did not appear until 7 – 8 days.

Variables	**Group of calves**		**P**
	Healthy (n = 15)	**Sick (n = 27)**	
Hp (mg/ml)	0.05 ± 0.06	1.11 ± 0.80	< 0.001
SAA (μg/ml)	28.02 ± 20.60	63.19 ± 39.42	< 0.01

P – significance of the differences in measured values between healthy and sick animals, n. s. – non significant

Table 2. Concentrations of Hp, and SAA in healthy animals and calves suffering from chronic respiratory diseases (mean ± SD) [72]

According to Nikunen et al. [75], the use of different acute phase proteins as markers of naturally occuring respiratory diseases is somewhat controversial. In the study presented by these authors, only *Pasteurella multocida* infection was associated with markedly increased concentrations of acute phase proteins. Similarly, Svensson et al. [76] concluded that the discriminative ability of serum Hp concentrations for indicating the clinical respiratory-tract disease in calves under field conditions is overall poor, and no better than rectal temperature. The usefulness of acute phase proteins for determining the response to therapy and making the right treatment decisions was evaluated by Carter et al. [77]. They found higher Hp concentrations in calves requiring more than one treatment compared to calves with one treatment. In addition, Berry et al. [78] showed that Hp concentrations are useful tool for predicting the number of antimicrobial treatments required in newly received feedlot calves.

The ability of acute phase proteins to clearly identify the calves with bronchopneumonia that would have required an anti-inflammatory treatment was investigated also by Humblet et al. [79]. The results presented by these authors showed that haptoglobin and fibrinogen together in growing calves suffering from bronchopneumonia allow the identification of about 70 % of calves that required antibiotic and anti-inflammatory drugs. Haptoglobin alone was able to confirm > 75 % of case decisions, whether diseased calves were treated or not. Moreover, Hp and Fbg were useful predictors of the inflammation severity. Jawor and Stefaniak [80] evaluated selected acute phase proteins and their usefulness as parameters for monitoring the treatment of respiratory diseases in calves. According to the aforementioned authors, the decreasing concentrations of acute phase proteins observed in the majority of calves treated for bronchopneumonia suggest diminishing inflammatory processes. In contrast, higher acute phase protein concentrations after an initial decrease strongly suggest the presence of secondary infections, meening that treatment should be continued.

Variables	**Group of sick calves**		**P**
	A (n = 16)	**B (n = 11)**	
Hp (mg/ml)	0.81 ± 0.60	1.56 ± 0.86	< 0.05
SAA (μg/ml)	44.70 ± 30.78	90.07 ± 35.73	< 0.01

Groups of calves: A – group of calves with improved general health state; B – group of died or euthanised calves

P – significance of the differences in measured values between two groups of sick calves, n. s. – non significant

Table 3. Comparison of the concentrations of Hp, and SAA between two groups of calves with respiratory-tract diseases, divided according to the development of their health status during the treatment (mean ± SD) [72]

Most of the investigations on the synthesis of acute phase proteins in animals with respiratory diseases have been focused on the immediate or acute phase response of the infection. However, only a few reports on the acute phase protein production in chronic inflammatory conditions have been published. Horadagoda et al. [18] found that the concentrations of Hp, SAA and α_1-acid glycoprotein were higher in cases of acute compared with chronic inflammation. The results presented by Tóthová et al. [72] showed that not only acute diseases of the respiratory tract, but also chronic cases are characterized with increased production of some acute phase proteins, predominantly haptoglobin with concentrations in calves with chronic respiratory diseases more than twentyfold higher compared with healthy animals (Table 2). In addition, in the aforementioned study, cases with severe clinical signs and poor prognosis were associated with markedly higher Hp and SAA concentrations (Table 3). Thus, Hp concentrations in the range of 1 – 3 mg/ml, and SAA concentrations around 100 μg/ml predict severe course of the disease with poor prognosis. Similar findings were reported in calves by Heegaard et al. [25]. Skinner et al. [81] found that Hp concentrations of more than 0.2 mg/ml indicate mild infection, values above 0.4 mg/ml suggest severe infection, while extended pathological conditions are typically associated with Hp values in the range of 1- 2 mg/ml. These results suggest the wide use and possible application of acute phase proteins to

http://dx.doi.org/10.5772/55857

determine respiratory diseases and the magnitude of inflammatory changes in calves, choose proper therapy and monitor the efficiency of the treatment.

7.1.2. Acute phase proteins in calves with diarrhoea

Diarrhoea in calves, together with respiratory diseases, is another multifactorial disease entity that can have serious financial and animal welfare implications in both dairy and beef suckler herds. It has been estimated that 75 % of early calf mortality in dairy herds is caused by diarrhoea in the pre-weaning period [82]. However, there are only few published data regarding the possible influence of diarrhoea on the concentrations of acute phase proteins and their usefulness in the diagnosis of these diseases. Piercy [83] investigated the production of ceruloplasmin in experimental infection with *Salmonella (S.) Dublin*. In the infected calves, they found a significant increase in the concentrations of ceruloplasmin between 3 and 4 days after infection, which decreased to normal values on day 7. Deignan et al. [84] examined the serum concentrations of haptoglobin, a more common bovine acute phase protein, in young calves in response to experimental infection with a mixture of three *Salmonella* serotypes (S. Dublin, S. enteritidis, S. Heidelberg), and to compare these levels with clinical markers of infection to assess the usefulness of Hp as a marker of infection severity. In the aforementioned study, the serum Hp concentrations prior to bacterial challenge were undetectable in all animals included in the trial. Following experimental *Salmonella* infection, the Hp concentrations increased significantly within 3 days of challenge. This increase in serum Hp values showed a statistical correlation with other more subjective clinical markers of infection, such as diarrhoeal scores, morbidity scores and temperature. On day 5 post-challenge, the serum Hp concentrations in *Salmonella*–challenged calves had returned to the normal values in all animals analyzed, despite the persistence of clinical symptoms of infection in the most of these animals. These obtained data indicate that Hp concentrations reflect the severity of infection, and may aid in predicting the prognosis of the infection. Similarly, Skinner et al. [81] indicated the significance of Hp as a clinically useful parameter for measuring the occurrence of enteritis in cattle.

The usefulness of the assessment of Hp, SAA and fibrinogen concentrations for the monitoring of treatment in calves having diarrhoea was evaluated by Jawor [85]. In the aforementioned study, 40 % of calves with diarrhoea had Hp concentration > 0.1 mg/ml (ranging to 0.49 mg/ml). During the treatment, the serum concentrations of Hp decreased. A high percentage of diarrhoeic calves with higher Fbg concentrations (mean Fbg concentration of 7.28 g/l) were detected at the beginning of the treatment, while during the treatment a gradual decrease was noted. However, fibrinogen estimation required an additional determination of plasma proteins to distinguish between a relative increase in hemoconcentration and an absolute increase of Fbg concentration during inflammation [53]. The concentrations of SAA were elevated during the entire treatment period for most of the diarrhoeic calves. The very high initial serum SAA concentrations and subsequent significant decrease of values during the treatment suggest that this acute phase protein may be very useful in calves with diarrhoea. Similarly, the results presented by Tóthová et al. [86] showed in 10 calves with clinical signs of diarrhoea higher mean SAA concentration compared with clinically healthy calves (Table

4). However, in Hp and Fbg concentrations they found no marked differences between healthy and diarrhoeic calves, and haptoglobin does not reach the concentrations seen in other disease conditions in cattle. Thus, these findings indicate that the disturbances in the homeostasis, inflammatory reactions of the organism, and tissue damage caused by diarrhoea did not evoke sufficient inflammatory response giving a more marked systemic increase in the concentrations of measured acute phase proteins. Similarly, according to Muller-Doblies et al. [87], Hp requires a stronger stimulation to induce an increase in serum concentrations.

Variables		**Groups of calves**					**K-W**
		H	**A**	**B**	**C**	**D**	***P***
Hp (mg/ml)	x	0.04[a]	0.73[a]	0.10	0.13	0.43	< 0.001
	SD	0.03	0.78	0.16	0.16	0.78	
SAA (μg/ml)	x	29.78[a]	93.38[a]	51.47	74.94	42.02	< 0.001
	SD	24.62	50.96	25.05	26.16	28.21	
Fbg (g/l)	x	2.31[a]	3.86[a]	2.84	2.81	3.16	< 0.001
	SD	0.41	1.55	0.77	0.51	1.22	

The same superscripts in rows mean statistical signif cance of differences in measured concentrations between the groups of calves: a – $P < 0.001$

K-W – Kruskal-Wallis analysis; P – significance of the analysis

Groups of calves: H – clinically healthy calves, A – calves with clinical signs of respiratory diseases, B – diarrhoeic calves, C – calves with omphalophlebitis, D – calves with multisystemic diseases

Table 4. Comparison of the concentrations of Hp, SAA and Fbg between clinically healthy calves and calves affected by various inflammatory diseases [86]

7.1.3. Acute phase proteins in calves with omphalophlebitis and multisystemic diseases

Seeing that the inflammation of the navel, the tissue damage and other pathologic lesions in the associated structures may cause inflammatory reactions, Tóthová et al. [86] evaluated calves with omphalophlebitis to detect if this disease may affect the concentrations of major acute phase proteins. The results presented in this study showed in calves with clinical signs of omphalophlebitis, similarly to the calves with diarrhoea, more markedly higher mean concentration of SAA than in clinically healthy calves. In the concentrations of Hp and Fbg there were no marked differences between healthy and sick animals (Table 4). These findings might be a consequence of a different initiation of the production of various acute phase proteins, seeing that SAA is a more sensitive acute phase protein than Hp in cattle, with rapid increase in serum concentrations after the inflammatory stimulus [88]. An opposite trend with more markedly higher mean concentrations of Hp and Fbg was observed by Tóthová et al. [86] in calves affected by multisystemic diseases (with more than one affected organ – navel, joints, digestive tract, respiratory system), while the mean SAA concentration obtained in this group was only slightly higher compared with clinically healthy calves. Similar findings were reported by Gänheim et al. [89], who found higher concentrations of Hp and fibrinogen in calves with diarrhoea at the same time as respiratory symptoms compared to those that had signs of only respiratory diseases or diarrhoea.

7.2. Acute phase proteins in dairy cows

7.2.1. Acute phase proteins in cows with mastitis

Despite world-wide efforts, mastitis has remained economically the most important disease in dairy cattle, and despite different mastitis control programs it is still the major challenge for the dairy industry [90]. While clinical mastitis is often easy to detect, sub-clinical mastitis, on the other hand, is a larger problem for the dairy industry since this condition shows no visible changes in the udder or in the milk [91]. Sub-clinical mastitis is frequently diagnosed by Californian Mastitis Test (CMT), which may suffer from a lack of reproducibility. In addition, up to now, the evaluation of somatic cell count (SCC) has remained as the gold standard for determining udder health. However, it is not sufficient enough in discriminating between the clinical and sub-clinical form of mastitis [92]. Therefore, it is of great importance to investigate biomarkers that could be used for rapid detection of sub-clinical mastitis. One of the ways to identify cows with sub-clinical mastitis would be the measuring of the concentrations of acute phase proteins. The production and usefulness of acute phase proteins in cows with experimentally induced mastitis and mastitis under field conditions were investigated by several authors.

Conner et al. [93] evaluated the concentrations of haptoglobin, ceruloplasmin and α-1 antitrypsin in cows with summer mastitis (septic mastitis) and clinically healthy cows. In all cows with mastitis, they found elevated concentrations of Hp, whereas in healthy cows the Hp values were undetectable. Moreover, all cows with summer mastitis included into this study had significantly higher concentrations of ceruloplasmin and α-1 antitrypsin in comparison to cows without mastitis. Skinner et al. [81] concluded that Hp concentrations of 0.2 g/l and above in cows with mastitis may indicate early or mild infection, while values higher than 0.4 g/l indicate severe infection.

The usefulness of acute phase proteins in the diagnosis of mastitis was investigated by Hirvonen et al. [94] in pregnant heifers experimentally infected with *Actinomyces pyogenes, Fusobacterium necrophorum* and *Peptostreptococcus indolicus*. They evaluated also the prognostic value of selected acute phase proteins (haptoglobin, fibrinogen, acid-soluble glycoproteins and α_1-proteinase inhibitor) in the infected animals. According to the aforementioned authors, fibrinogen was a reliable indicator for detecting the presence of bacterial infection in all heifers, but not as a prognostic indicator for mastitis, as they found no significant differences in the production of Fbg between animals which recovered and those without response to treatment. They indicated Hp and acid-soluble glycoproteins as the most effective markers in the determination of the severity of infection and in predicting the final outcome of the disease in heifers with mastitis. The concentrations of Hp increased significantly in the infected heifers with the maximum values reached after 2 – 3 days after inoculation. However, the Hp response was different between moderate and severely affected animals. Hirvonen et al. [94] reported that in severely infected heifers, the concentrations of Hp were four times higher than in the moderately affected heifers, and these values remained elevated 2 weeks after bacterial inoculation. On the other hand, in the moderately affected heifers, haptoglobin returned to normal values 5 days after the bacterial challenge. In a later study, Hirvonen et al. [95] examined the changes in some acute phase proteins in cows with acute experimental *Escherichia (E.) coli* mastitis and their role in predicting the outcome from the disease. The cows included into this study were challenged with 1500 cfu of *E. coli* FT238 strain into one udder quarter, and 3 weeks later into the contralateral quarter. In the aforementioned study, the intramammary infection with *E.coli* produced a clinical mastitis and induced an increase in the serum Hp and SAA concentrations in all cows. The concentrations of Hp were normalized within 7 days, and SAA values by the 6th day after inoculation. In addition, these authors found that the differences between severely versus moderately or mildly affected cows with *E. coli* were present for SAA, but not for Hp. The concentrations of SAA were related to the severity of the disease; in cows with fatal mastitis the SAA concentrations progressively rose. Thus, serum amyloid A appeared to be a promising indicator for the course of *E. coli* mastitis. Similar findings were reported by Eckersall et al. [96] in cows with clinical mastitis (bacteria isolated including *E. coli, Staphylococcus aureus, Streptococcus uberis, Streptococcus dysgalactiae* and *Arcanobacter pyogenes*). They found significantly higher serum concentrations of Hp, as well as SAA in cows with both mild and moderate mastitis compared to healthy cows. However, these authors observed no significant differences between the cows suffering from mild and moderate mastitis.

The hypothesis that the major acute phase proteins in cows may be transferred into milk during the acute phase response caused by mastitis was investigated by adapting the assays to measure the concentrations of proteins in milk. Eckersall et al. [96] reported also that the most of serum proteins leak into milk across the blood-mammary barrier as a result of the disruption caused by the inflammation due to mastitis. Moreover, milk seems to be a better sample material than serum for testing the concentrations of acute phase proteins during mastitis (easier and quicker sample collection without stressing the animals). The potential value of measuring the concentrations of acute phase proteins in milk as a means of detecting mastitis in cows was assessed by Eckersall et al. [96]. According to their results, the milk samples from cows with both mild and moderate mastitis had significantly higher Hp, as well as SAA concentrations than the milk from healthy cows. Moreover, in milk samples from cows with moderate mastitis, the SAA concentrations were significantly higher than in cows with mild mastitis. On the other hand, in the milk Hp concentrations there were no significant differences between the infected cows. Thus, the milk SAA concentrations seem to have a greater potential for the detection of the severity of mastitis, since it has higher sensitivity and specificity in differentiating cows with mastitis [96].

The SAA response in milk and plasma to experimental intramammary inoculation of *E. coli* in cows was examined by Jacobsen et al. [97]. In this study, plasma and milk samples were obtained from cows before and after intramammary inoculation with 50 cfu of a non-verotoxic encapsulated strain of *E. coli* O:157. Prior to inoculation, the plasma and milk samples had no or very low concentrations of serum amyloid A. All cows, regardless of the severity of infection, showed elevated SAA concentrations in milk and plasma after inoculation. Milk SAA concentrations began to increase between 6 and 12 hours after inoculation (approximately 80

http://dx.doi.org/10.5772/55857

times), and plasma SAA values increased between 12 and 24 hours *post inoculation*. The rapid increase in milk concentrations after intramammary inoculation of mastitis pathogens suggests that SAA may be particularly suited for early detection of mastitis [98]. The fast return towards baseline values after bacterial clearance suggests that milk SAA measurements may also be used as indicators of treatment efficiency. In the study presented by Jacobsen et al. [97], cows with severe mastitis had a particularly increased milk SAA concentrations at 48 hours after inoculation, which stayed elevated throughout the study period. In cows with moderate and mild mastitis, milk SAA values started to decrease at 60 and 48 hours after inoculation, respectively. As cows with severe mastitis had higher milk SAA concentrations than cows with moderate or mild mastitis, SAA may therefore serve as an indicator of the degree of tissue damage and hence prognosis and expected production loss during episodes of mastitis. Higher concentrations of Hp and SAA in serum and milk of cows with clinical mastitis were observed also by Nielsen et al. [99]. In addition, these authors concluded that the concentrations of acute phase proteins in milk significantly increased with increasing somatic cell count, which suggest that these protein may indicate the severity of the infection.

Grönlund et al. [100] examined the concentrations of Hp and SAA in cows with naturally occuring chronic sub-clinical mastitis. The comparison of acute phase protein concentrations in quarter and composite milk samples was made also in this study. Almost all quarter milk samples from healthy control cows had undetectable concentrations of Hp and SAA. In cows with chronic sub-clinical mastitis, increased concentrations of both measured acute phase proteins in milk were observed, indicating an activation of the acute phase response also in cows with chronic mastitis, but the contents of Hp and SAA varied markedly. Haptoglobin and SAA were detected by the aforementioned authors in 83 % of the examined composite milk samples. Thus, according to Grönlund et al. [100], since cows had to have detectable concentrations of Hp or SAA in at least two udder quarters for elevated values to be found in the composite samples, analysis at the quarter level is preferable.

Further investigations showed an extrahepatic synthesis of specific isoform of serum amyloid A directly from mammary epithelial cells (M-SAA) [32]. Therefore, M-SAA is believed to be more sensitive indicator of mastitis, which accumulates in milk only during mammary inflammation. The usefulness of M-SAA in the diagnosis of clinical and sub-clinical mastitis in cows with various clinical findings on the mammary gland was investigated by Kováč et al. [101]. Their results showed markedly higher M-SAA concentrations in milk samples from quarters with clinical changes, as well as from quarters without clinical signs of mastitis, but with strongly positive Californian Mastitis Test (Table 5). In addition, the concentrations of M-SAA found in samples from mammary quarters without clinical changes were also relatively high (mean value of 473.7 ng/ml), as the uninfected mammary quarters had to have very low or undetectable concentrations of M-SAA. These results suggest that some quarters might be affected by inflammatory process, but still without positive reaction of CMT. Elevated concentrations of M-SAA in quarters with mastitis compared to healthy quarters were reported also by Petersen et al. [102] and Nazifi et al. [103].

Variable		Groups of cows				K-W
		I. (n=7)	II. (n=12)	III. (n=13)	IV. (n=9)	P
M-SAA (ng/ml)	x	325.7[A,B]	1433.1[a]	3910.4[A]	6073.8[B,a]	< 0.001
	± SD	173.8	949.2	2145.8	4414.0	
Hp (mg/ml)	x	0.046	0.122	0.299	0.329	< 0.05
	± SD	0.053	0.263	0.314	0.339	
SAA (μg/ml)	x	29.7	27.6[a]	48.2	71.5[a]	< 0.05
	± SD	27.6	28.0	42.5	31.5	

The same superscripts in rows mean statistical significance of differences in measured concentrations between the groups of cows: a – $P < 0.05$; A, B – $P < 0.001$

K-W – Kruskal-Wallis analysis; P – significance of the analysis

Groups of cows: I – cows without clinical findings on the mammary gland and with negative CMT, II – cows without clinical findings on the mammary gland and with weakly positive CMT, III – cows without clinical findings on the mammary gland and with strongly positive CMT, IV – cows with clinical changes and changes in the milk appearance

Table 5. The concentrations of M-SAA, Hp, and SAA in dairy cows with various findings on the mammary gland [101]

The response characterized by increased synthesis of M-SAA is specific for the quarter and does not necessarily result in detectable concentrations in composite milk samples. The results presented by Kováč et al. [101] showed similar trend of changes in the concentrations of M-SAA in composite milk samples and in samples from separate quarters, but the values measured were lower in composite milk samples, which suggest a diluting effect of milk from quarters with less marked changes (Table 5). Grönlund et al. [100] reported also some interpretative problems by the use of composite milk samples if only one quarter is sub-clinically infected. Therefore, it seems that composite milk samples are less suitable for detection of sub-clinical mastitis than samples from separate mammary quarters. In addition, the results presented by Kováč et al. [101] showed in cows with clinical mastitis higher concentrations of Hp and SAA in blood serum (Table 5), which suggest that localized severe inflammation of the udder is sufficiently intense to induce a measurable systemic acute phase response. However, the finding that the differences in serum Hp and SAA concentrations observed between the groups of cows with various clinical findings on the mammary gland were less significant than the differences in M-SAA concentrations means that the measuring of serum concentrations of some acute phase proteins would be less useful to the evaluation of the severity of mastitis than the measuring of the concentrations of M-SAA directly in milk samples.

7.2.2. Acute phase proteins in cows after parturition and cows with peripartum reproductive disorders

The period after parturition is the most critical period in dairy cows regarding health status and production. Factors such as pregnancy, parturition, blood calcium concentrations, initiation of lactation and feed intake all affect the ability of the cow's immune system to effectively combat infections. The periparturient period is the time where these complex physiological changes occur simultaneously, having a significant effect on the animal's health [104]. Parturition, changes in homeostasis, metabolic and physiological challenges occuring in this stressful period, as well as other external and internal harmful stimuli may contribute to the activation of host immune system and inflammatory responses, including the initiation of the production of acute phase proteins. Major bovine acute phase proteins, haptoglobin and serum amyloid A, play an important role also in the reproductive processes, they intensify the phagocytosis process against the pathogens introduced into the uterus, and help by the reconstruction of the endometrium [105].

Saini et al. [106] reported that lactation and pregnancy in cattle appeared to have no effect on the Hp concentration in blood serum. However, according to Gymnich et al. [107] haptoglobin concentrations undergo significant changes around parturition, and in horses and cows the highest concentrations were observed 1 day post partum. Uchida et al. [108] evaluated the concentration of Hp in cows in the periparturient period and they observed significantly higher values around parturition than before and after parturition. Similarly, Ametaj [109] and Tóthová et al. [110] reported in cows after parturition an increase of two main acute phase proteins, Hp and SAA. According to the results presented by Chan et al. [111], the SAA concentrations in healthy cows reached the highest values within 3 days after the delivery (mean value of 66 mg/l). The Hp concentrations in the most of the evaluated animals were higher than 130.9 mg/l within 3 days after calving. Parturition with following metabolic challenges constitutes a potentially stressful event for the dairy cow. One of the ways how an animal can manifest stress is in the form of activated acute phase response, including the increased production of acute phase proteins by the liver. According to Alsemgeest et al. [112], the physiological processes taking place around the time of parturition are mainly responsible for higher concentrations of acute phase proteins in blood serum. Regassa and Noakes [113] reported that higher values of acute phase proteins could be related to the tissue damage occuring due to the increased myometrial activity during expulsion of the calf, involution of the uterus, as well as degeneration and regeneration of the endometrium. Young et al. [114] found that higher concentrations of these proteins, determined in the last phase of pregnancy and after calving may be connected with the changing hormone profile (the influence of estrogens and progesterone). In addition, it is worth pointing out that the increase in acute phase protein concentrations in cattle may be caused also by the increased concentrations of cortisol [115].

Postpartum endometritis is a common problem in cattle, because uterine contamination following calving is frequent, but most cows are able to eliminate bacteria from the uterus within 2 to 3 weeks after calving without manifesting marked clinical signs of the disease. However, cows that can not eliminate the infection may subsequently develop endometritis. Skinner et al. [81] reported that Hp concentrations are high in cows with metritis, with mean serum Hp concentration in cows with severe metritis of 1.04 g/l. Chan et al. [116] evaluated clinically healthy cows and cows with postpartum reproductive diseases after calving, and the Hp concentrations in clinically diseased cows (1133.5 mg/l) were significantly higher than in clinically healthy cows (104.6 mg/l). In a later study presented by Chan et al. [111], cows with acute puerperal metritis had significantly higher Hp concentrations than those in healthy cows throughout the

6 months after delivery. The highest Hp concentration was found in the period of 3 days after parturition (1.1 g/l), and for SAA concentrations 4 – 7 days *post partum* (85 mg/l). However, postpartum metritis does not necessarily need to be manifested by general clinical signs of the disease; frequently only subfertility and a decrease of the milk yield are found. Moreover, various cows with mild uterine inflammation are able to restore health spontaneously without more serious consequences. Low Hp concentrations were found by Smith et al. [117] in cows with toxic puerperal metritis. Hirvonen et al. [118] reported also that the Hp concentrations remained low or moderate in the most of cows with acute postpartum metritis. However, the data obtained in recent years suggest that acute phase proteins may be used as early predictors or risk factors for metritis. Huzzey et al. [119] showed that cows with Hp concentrations higher than 1 g/l at day 3 *post partum* were 6.7 times more likely to develop mild or severe metritis. Similarly, Dubuc et al. [120] concluded that Hp concentrations higher than 0.8 g/l in the first week after parturition are a risk factor for endometritis, as well as purulent vaginal discharge.

The usefulness of acute phase proteins by the evaluation of the efficiency of therapy was investigated by Mordak [121] in cows with retained placenta (with or without manual removal of the membrane). The highest Hp concentration they found in cows where the placenta had been expelled after 4 days (2.22 g/l), and the lowest in cows where the placenta had been easily removed manually (0.9 g/l).

7.2.3. Acute phase proteins in cows with hoof diseases and lameness

Bovine lameness and hoof diseases represent one of the major health problems for the dairy industry, and raise important questions about economic aspects and welfare issues in agriculture [122]. Economic losses arise from decreased milk production, poor performance, fertility problems, increasing culling rates and treatment costs. The predominant hoof problems causing lameness in cows are sole ulcers, white line abscesses, interdigital phlegmons and digital dermatitis [123]. Disorders in the locomotory system (due to damaged tissues, painfull processes, impaired homeostasis) may lead to a systemic acute phase response characterized by higher concentrations of some acute phase proteins. Therefore, some acute phase proteins may be useful in the early detection of lame cows in order to limit the losses related to lameness.

Variables	**Groups of animals**		**P**
	Healthy (n = 23)	**Sick (n = 35)**	
Hp (mg/ml)	0.094 ± 0.086	0.450 ± 0.601	< 0.05
SAA (µg/ml)	12.70 ± 16.80	113.90 ± 55.66	< 0.001
Fbg (g/l)	2.19 ± 0.37	2.95 ± 0.65	< 0.001

P – significance of the differences in measured values between healthy and sick animals, n. s. – non significant

Table 6. Comparison of the concentrations of evaluated acute phase proteins in healthy animals and heifers with hoof diseases (mean ± SD) [125]

The usefulness of acute phase proteins in the detection of lame cows was evaluated by Kujala et al. [124]. They investigated the acute phase response, including the concentrations of Hp and SAA in cows with sole ulcers and white line diseases. Their results showed higher concentrations of SAA in lame cows than in healthy animals, with values elevated from day 0 until days 7 – 8. The SAA concentrations started to decrease on day 14. In the serum Hp concentrations, no significant differences between healthy and lame cows were found. Significantly higher concentrations of Hp, SAA, as well as fibrinogen were found by Tóthová et al. [125] in heifers with hoof diseases (including pododermatitis, laminitis, sole ulcer, and digital dermatitis) compared to healthy animals (Table 6). Laven et al. [126] evaluated the concentrations of Hp, Fbg, ceruloplasmin and seromucoid in first lactation heifers with hoof horn haemoorhagies to determine the relationships with the development of the disease. However, they found any relationships between the presence of acute phase response and the development of hoof horn haemorrhagies in heifers after calving.

The presence of acute phase response in association with lameness due to claw disorders was investigated by Smith et al. [127] in dairy cattle on a commercial farm. In addition, they evaluated the effect of treatment on the acute phase protein concentrations and thus measured the effectiveness of the treatment. Into the evaluation they included cows diagnosed with pododermatitis septica, pododermatitis circumscripta, interdigital necrobacillosis and papillomatosis, digital dermatitis, as well healthy cows as control animals. The concentrations of serum Hp of all healthy cows without lameness were undetectable. Lame cows with any of the presented claw disorders were found to have increased serum Hp concentrations. In animals with pododermatitis septica and interdigital necrobacillosis, the Hp concentrations decreased after the treatment between days 1 to 5, which indicated effective treatment for these disorders. In contrast, treatment did not affect the concentrations of Hp in animals with pododermatitis circumscripta. Jawor et al. [128] evaluated the concentrations of acute phase proteins at selected time points during the treatment of cows with limb diseases with an aid to monitor the treatment and as an early predivtive marker of possible complications. In the examined cows, arthritis, sole ulcer, and white line disease were the most often diagnosed diseases. The highest concentrations of Hp, SAA and Fbg were recorded at the beginning of the treatment. In the cows, in which the treatment process went without complications, a high gradual decrease of acute phase protein concentrations was observed. This proved that the treatment applied was appropriate and that it contributed towards reducing the inflammatory process in cows. In cows with further complications (e.g. wound infections, bronchitis, the occurence of other inflammatory states of the limbs), they found increases in one or two of the measured acute phase proteins at the next blood collection. This indicates that these cows had not completely recovered and the treatment should be continued.

7.2.4. Acute phase proteins in cows with abdominal disorders

The usefulness of the measurement of acute phase protein concentrations in cattle, predominantly of fibrinogen, has been described in traumatic pericarditis, reticuloperitonitis, abomasal displacement, and by the monitoring of postoperative complications, as well as by the differentiation of reticuloperitonitis from other gastrointestinal disorders [51,129]. Very high plasma Fbg concentrations were reported by McSherry et al. [130] in cows with pericarditis and peritonitis.

After abdominal surgery, the condition of the patient is usually followed-up by physical observation. As complications are frequent, a more accurate indicator of their occurrence and severity would be valuable. Therefore, Hirvonen and Pyörälä [51] evaluated the usefulness of Fbg and Hp in the diagnosis of traumatic reticuloperitonitis in dairy cows. In addition, they studied how abdominal surgery affects these parameters, and whether they can be used to predict recovery from abdominal disorders. In this study, the preoperative Fbg and Hp concentrations in cows with traumatic reticuloperitonitis were significantly higher than those for cows with abomasal displacement or explorative laparotomy. The plasma Fbg values in cows with traumatic reticuloperitonitis remained high for about 2 days after surgery. The Hp concentrations in these cows showed only a small increase, which was followed by a steady decrease during the late hospitalization phase. However, the concentrations of both Fbg and Hp remained above normal values at the time of hospital discharge. Moreover, the values measured correlated well with the clinical findings from those cows with traumatic reticuloperitonitis. Thus, Hirvonen and Pyörälä [51] concluded that these proteins may be attractive parameters for the evaluation in the diagnostic of traumatic reticuloperitonitis.

According to McSherry et al. [130], displacement of the abomasum does not usually induce a significant fibrinogen response. In the study presented by Jawor et al. [131] the Fbg concentrations in cows with displaced abomasum were within normal values. Significant changes during the post-operative monitoring were found only for SAA concentrations. Nazifi et al. [132] evaluated the possible relationships between cardiac diseases (functional murmurs, pathologic murmurs, endocarditis, and pericarditis) and the concentrations of acute phase proteins in dairy cattle. In this study, cases with pericarditis and endocarditis had higher Hp and SAA concentrations than the cows with functional and pathological murmurs. In addition, the concentrations of the both measured acute phase proteins were lower in cows with endocarditis than those measured in cows with pericarditis, which suggest that the measurement of acute phase proteins can be helpful in differentiating an acute inflammatory condition like pericarditis from other cardiac disorders.

8. Acute phase proteins in swine diseases

Acute phase protein testing offers a tool for assessing a health status also in pig production systems. An important practical aspect in the pig production is the sub-clinical condition that does not lead to overt disease but may cause suboptimal growth and decreased welfare. A number of investigations indicate the ability of acute phase protein measurements to reveal such conditions [133,15]. In addition, lower gaining pigs were found to have higher acute phase protein levels than high gaining pigs [134].

Porcine C-reactive protein has been found to rise in experimental models of *Mycoplasma hyorhinis, Toxoplasma gondii, Actinobacillus pleuropneumoniae* and porcine reproductive and respiratory syndrome virus infection [135]. Sorensen et al. [136] evaluated the acute phase response in the pigs experimentally infected with *Streptococcus (S.) suis* serotype 2. Already on day 1 after inoculation, the CRP concentrations increased sharply in all animals and in general reached the maximum values between days 1 and 5 after infection, showing an approximately 10-fold increase as compared to initial values. From around day 8 *post inoculation*, the response started to decrease. The SAA concentrations rose sharply in all pigs on day 1 after infection with *S.suis.*, and peaked already on days 1 and 2, reaching peak levels of at least 30–40 times the values before infection. Regarding the Hp concentrations, its values increased from the day 1 after inoculation in all animals, but increase was less marked compared to CRP and SAA. In addition, the acute phase response following inoculation with *S. suis* was closely correlated with the clinical signs and pathological lesions typical to *S. suis* infection. Thus, Sorensen et al. [136] concluded the usefulness of acute phase proteins in the detection of ongoing *S. suis* infection. The usefulness of serum haptoglobin in the determination of progressive atrophic rhinitis in pigs was evaluated by Francisco et al. [137]. They investigated the serum Hp concentrations in growing swine after intranasal challenge with varying doses of *Pasteurella (P.) multocida* type D (toxigenic strain) and *Bordetella (B.) bronchiseptica*. While increasing doses of *P. multocida* tended to increase serum Hp concentrations, increasing the dose of *B. bronchiseptica* was associated with reduced Hp values in this model. Significant positive correlations of the Hp concentrations and atrophic rhinitis scores were found by the aforementioned authors, indicating that increased serum haptoglobin is associated with higher incidences of atrophic rhinitis in swine. Quereda et al. [138] investigated the diagnostic value of acute phase proteins in the determination of pig infectious wasting diseases. They evaluated pigs from farms in which postweaning multisystemic wasting syndrome (PMWS) and porcine respiratory disease complex (PRDC) were diagnosed. In this study, serum Hp concentrations were significantly higher in pigs with PMWS and PRDC than in the specific pathogen free pigs. The serum CRP and SAA concentrations were significantly higher in pigs with PMWS than in healthy pigs. However, there were no significant differences for these proteins between healthy and PRDC pigs. In addition, Quereda et al. [138] concluded that CRP and SAA could be used as a complementary tool to monitor the existence of lymphoid depletion, and Hp could provide information about the severity of this depletion.

The relationships between the serum concentrations of acute phase proteins and the appearance and severity of lesions in pigs at slaughter was evaluated by Pallarés et al. [139]. They determined whether the concentrations of acute phase proteins could be used as markers for the presence of lesions and as a tool to detect sub-clinical disease in fattening pigs. In the aforementioned study, the concentrations of CRP in pigs with clinical signs of diseases and poor body condition were significantly higher than in apparently healthy pigs with gross lesions at slaughter (about 2.1 fold higher) and in apparently healthy pigs without gross lesions at slaghter (about 2.5 higher). Moreover, they found significant differences between apparently healthy pigs with marked lesions and without marked lesions at slaughter. Similar findings were recorded also in the serum Hp concentrations. For the concentrations of SAA, although the values recorded in pigs with clinical diseases were significantly higher than in apparently healthy pigs, the differences between pigs with gross lesions and without gross lesions were not significant. In addition, the serum CRP concentrations were significantly higher in pigs showing lesions in the lungs and one or more other organs compared to pigs showing lesions only in the lungs. Thus, the results presented by Pallarés et al. [139] indicate that the serum concentrations of CRP, SAA, as well as Hp can be used as markers of clinical diseases in pigs. These findings agree with those of Chen et al. [140], in which serum Hp and CRP concentrations were significantly higher in culled pigs than in clinically healthy pigs. However, according to Pallarés et al. [139], only Hp and CRP could be used as markers of the presence of lesions at slaughter, since they appear to differentiate apparently healthy pigs with lesions from pigs with no lesions. The presence of elevated serum Hp and CRP concentrations in apparently healthy pigs at slaughter could provide important information to a veterinary inspector about the presence of sub-clinical lesions that could lead to condemnations or a decrease in the quality of carcasses.

9. Conclusion

The objective determination of animal health is important due to the increasing focus of consumers and farmers on the welfare of animals. As non-specific markers of inflammation, acute phase protein testing is a useful tool for the assessment of health in general, to monitor the health state, the spread of infection or the efficacy of treatment. The measurement of acute phase proteins may also be useful in defining the objective health status of an animal or a herd. They are reliable biomarkers that can be used both in diagnostic approaches and for research purposes.

Practical uses and advantages of acute phase protein assays have been described in a large number of scientific reports published in the last few years. Clinical application of acute phase proteins has not been extensive in routine clinical animal practice due to practical limitations associated with their analysis. The most of the methods available for measuring specific acute phase proteins are immunological methods, which are time-consuming and relatively expensive, so limiting the wide-scale use of acute phase proteins in routine practice. Seeing that there is a broad spectrum of possible applications of acute phase protein based diagnostics for the use in ruminants and swine, it is necessary to develop and optimise rapid field tests that allow the determination of acute phase proteins in a short time period.

Despite the challenges in the determination of acute phase proteins, with the insights provided by ongoing research in this area, it is likely that these analytes will be increasingly used in the diagnosis and prognosis of diseases also in farm animal medicine. Acute phase proteins have proven to be very useful in the early detection of sub-clinical diseases or alterations of the health status of an animal, with predictive information regarding the development of disease. Changes in the serum concentrations of acute phase proteins indicate the need for a more detailed clinical evaluation of a patient. In addition, acute phase proteins can be a powerful tool in the monitoring of treatment.

Acknowledgements

This work was supported by VEGA Scientific Grants No 1/0592/12 and 1/0812/12 from the Ministry of Education, and by Slovak Research and Development Agency under contract No. APVV-0475-10.

Author details

Csilla Tóthová, Oskar Nagy and Gabriel Kováč

*Address all correspondence to: tothova@uvm.sk

Clinic for Ruminants, University of Veterinary Medicine and Pharmacy, Košice, Slovak Republic

References

[1] Murata H., Shimada N., Yoshioka M. Current research on acute phase proteins in veterinary diagnosis: an overview. The Veterinary Journal 2004; 168: 28-40.

[2] Baumann H., Gauldie J. The acute phase response. Immunology Today 1994; 15: 74-80.

[3] Johnson HL., Chiou CC., Cho CT. Applications of acute phase reactants in infectious diseases. Journal of Microbiology, Immunology, Infection 1999; 32: 73-82.

[4] Whicher T., Bienvenu J., Price CP. Molecular biology, measurement and clinical utility of the acute phase proteins. Pure and Applied Chemistry 1991; 63 (8): 1111-1116.

[5] Endre ZH., Westhuyzen J. Early detection of acute kidney injury: emerging new biomarkers. Nephrology (Carlton) 2008; 13: 91-98.

[6] Cray C., Zaias J., Altman NH. Acute phase response in animals: a review. Comparative Medicine 2009; 59 (6): 517-526.

[7] Fearon DT., Locksley RM. The instructive role of innate imunity in the acquired immune response. Science 1996; 272: 50-54.

[8] Janeway CA., Travers P., Walport M., Schlomschik MJ. Immunobiology. 5th ed., London: Taylor & Francis; 2001.

[9] Bochsler PN., Slauson DO. Inflammation and repair of tissue. In: Bochcler PN:, Slauson DO. (eds.). Mechanism of disease. A textbook of comparative general pathology. 3rd ed., St. Louis: Mosby; 2002. p140-245.

[10] Moshage H. Cytokines and the hepatic acute phase response. Journal of Pathology 1997; 181: 257-266.

[11] Gabay C., Kushner I. Acute-phase proteins and other systemic responses to inflammation. New England Journal of Medicine 1999; 340: 448-454.

[12] Gruys E., Toussaint MJM., Niewold TA., Koopmans SJ. Acute phase reaction and acute phase proteins. Journal of Zhejiang University Science 2005; 6B (11): 1045-1056.

[13] Pyörälä S. Hirvonen's thesis on acute phase response in dairy cattle. PhD thesis. University of Helsinki, Helsinki, Finnland, ISBN 951-45-9104-6; 2000.

[14] Raynes JG. The acute phase response. Biochemical Society Transactions 1994; 22: 69-74.

[15] Petersen HH., Nielsen JP., Heegaard PMH. Application of acute phase protein measurements in veterinary clinical chemistry. Veterinary Research 2004; 35: 136-187.

[16] Cerón JJ., Eckersall PD., Martinez-Subiela S. Acute phase proteins in dogs and cats: current knowledge and future perspectives. Veterinary Clinical Pathology 2005; 34: 85-99.

[17] Niewold TA., Toussaint MJM., Gruys E. Monitoring health by acute phase proteins. Proceedings of the Fourth European Colloquium on Acute Phase Proteins. Segovia, Spain; 2003, p57-67.

[18] Horadagoda NU., Knox KM., Gibbs HA., Reid SW., Horadagoda A., Edwards SE., Eckersall PD. Acute phase proteins in cattle: Discrimination between acute and chronic inflammation. Veterinary Record 1999; 144: 437–441.

[19] Ceciliani F., Giordano A., Spagnolo V. The systemic reaction during inflammation: the acute phase proteins. Protein and Peptide Letters 2002; 9: 211-223.

[20] Wagener FA., Eggernt A., Boerman OC., Oyen WJ., Verhofstad A., Abraham NG., Adema G., van Kooyk Y., de Witte T., Figdor CG. Heme is a potent inducer of inflammation in mice and is countected by heme oxygenase. Blood 2002; 98: 1802-1811.

[21] Rossbacher J., Wagner L., Pasternack MS. Inhibitory effect of haptoglobin on granulocyte chemotaxis, phagocytosis and bactericidal activity. Scandinavian Journal of Immunology 1999; 50: 399-404.

[22] Eckersall PD., Bell R. Acute phase proteins: Biomarkers of infection and inflammation in veterinary medicine. The Veterinary Journal 2010; 185: 23-27.

[23] Lampreave F., Gonzalez-Ramon N., Martinez-Ayensa S., Hernandez M-A., Lorenzo H-K., Garcia-Gil A., Pineiro A. Characterisation of the acute phase serum protein response in pigs. Electrophoresis 1994; 15: 672-676.

[24] Kent J. Acute phase proteins: their use in veterinary diagnosis. British Veterinary Journal 1992; 148: 279-281.

[25] Heegaard PMH., Godson DL., Toussaint MJM., Tjornehoj K., Larsen LE., Viuff B., Ronsholt L. The acute phase response of haptoglobin and serum amyloid A (SAA) in cattle undergoing experimental infection with bovine respiratory syncytial virus. Veterinary Immunology and Immunopathology 2000; 77: 151-159.

[26] Bittrich S., Philipona C., Hammon HM., Romé V., Guilloteau P., Blum JW. Preterm as compared with full-term neonatal calves are characterized by morphological and

functional immaturity of the small intestine. Journal of Dairy Science 2004; 87: 1786-1795.

[27] Odle J. New insights into the utilization of medium-chain triglycerides by the neonate: observation from a piglet model. Journal of Nutrition 1997; 127: 1061-1067.

[28] Orro T., Jacobsen S., LePage J-P., Niewold T., Alasuutari S., Soveri T. Temporal changes in serum concentrations of acute phase proteins in newborn dairy calves. The Veterinary Journal 2008; 176: 182-187.

[29] Morein B., Abusugra I., Blomquist G. Immunity in neonates. Veterinary Immunology and Immunopathology 2002; 87: 207-213.

[30] Yamanaka H., Hagiwara K., Kirisawa R., Iwai H. Transient detection of proinflammatory cytokines in sera of colostrum-fed newborn calves. Journal of Veterinary Medical Science 2003; 65: 813-816.

[31] Schroedl W., Jaekel L., Krueger M. C-reactive protein and antibacterial activity in blood plasma of colostrum-fed calves and the effect of lactulose. Journal of Dairy Science 2003; 86: 3313-3320.

[32] McDonald TL., Larson MA., Mack DR., Weber A. Elevated extrahepatic expression and secretion of mammary-associated serum amyloid A 3 (M-SAA3) into colostrum. Veterinary Immunology and Immunopathology 2001; 83: 203-211.

[33] Dobryszycka W. Biological functions of haptoglobin, new pieces to an old puzzle. European Journal of Clinical Chemistry and Clinical Biochemistry 1997; 35: 647-654.

[34] Tóthová Cs., Nagy O., Seidel H., Kováč G. Age-related changes in the concentrations of acute phase proteins and some variables of protein metabolism in calves. Wiener Tierärztliche Monatschrift – Veterinary Medicine Austria 2011; 98: 33-44.

[35] Alsemgeest SPM., Jonker FH., Taverne MAM., Kalsbeek HC., Wensing T., Gruys E. Serum amyloid A and haptoglobin plasma concentrations in newborn calves. Theriogenology 1995; 43: 381-387.

[36] Hyvönen P., Suojala L., Orro T., Haaranen J., Simola O., Rontved C., Pyörälä S. Transgenic cows that produce recombinant human lactoferrin in milk are not protected from experimental *Escherichia coli* intramammary infection. Infection and Immunity 2006; 74: 6206-6212.

[37] Knowles TG., Edwards JE.. Bazeley KJ., Brown SN., Butterworth A., Warriss PD. Changes in the blood biochemical and haematological profile in neonatal calves with age. Veterinary Record 2000; 18: 593-598.

[38] Gentry PA., Ross ML., Hayatgheybi H. Competency of blood coagulation in the newborn calf. Research in Veterinary Science 1994; 57: 336-342.

[39] Morimatsu M., Syuto B., Shimada N., Fujinaga T., Yamamoto S., Saito M., Naiki M. Isolation and characterisation of bovine haptoglobin from acute phase sera. Journal of Biological Chemistry 1991; 266: 11833-11837.

[40] Godson DL., Campos M., Attah-Poku SK., Redmond MJ., Cordeiro DM., Sethi MS., Harland RJ., Babiuk LA. Serum haptoglobin as an indicator of the acute phase response in bovine respiratory disease. Veterinary Immunology and Immunopathology 1996; 51: 277-302.

[41] Yang FM., Haile DJ., Berger FG., Herbert DC., Van Beveren E., Ghio AJ. Haptoglobin reduces lung injury associated with exposure to blood. American Journal of Physiology and Lung Cell Molecular Physiology 2003; 284: L402-L409.

[42] Eckersall PD. Measurement of acute phase proteins as biomarkers of disease in production animals. Proceedings of the 57th Annual Meeting of the American College of Veterinary Pathologists and the 41st Annual Meeting of the American Society for Veterinary Clinical Pathology, 2-6 December 2006, Tucson, Arizona, USA; 2006. www.ivis.org (accessed March 2008)

[43] Makimura S., Suzuki N. Quantitative determination of bovine serum haptoglobin and its elevation in some inflammatory diseases. Japanese Journal of Veterinary Science 1982; 44: 15-21.

[44] Eckersall PD., Duthie S., Safi S., Moffatt D., Horadagoda NU., Doyle S, Parton R., Bennett D., Fitzpatrick JL. An automated biochemical assay for haptoglobin: Prevention of interference from albumin. Comparative Haematology International 1999; 5: 117-124.

[45] Weidmeyer CE., Solter PF. Validation of human haptoglobin immunoturbidimetric detection of haptoglobin in equine and canine serum and plasma. Veterinary Clinical Pathology 1996; 25: 141-146.

[46] Jensen LE., Whitehead AS. Regulation of serum amyloid A protein expression during the acute phase response. Biochemical Journal 1998; 334: 489-503.

[47] Weber A., Weber AT., McDonald TL., Larson MA. *Staphylococcus aureus* lipotechoic acid induces differential expression of bovine serum amyloid A3 (SAA3) by mammary epithelial cells: Implications of early diagnosis of mastitis. Veterinary Immunology and Immunopathology 2006; 109: 79-83.

[48] Mack DR., McDonald TL., Larson MA., Wei S., Weber A. The conserved TFLK motif of mammary-associated serum amyloid A is responsible for up-regulation of intestinal MUC3 mucin expression *in vitro*. Pediatric Research 2003; 53: 137-142.

[49] Yamamoto S., Miyadi S., Ashida Y. Preparartion of anti-canine serum amyloid A (SAA) serum and purification of SAA from canine high-density lipoprotein. Veterinary Immunology and Immunopathology 1994; 41: 41-53.

[50] Stoneham SJ., Palmer L., Cash R., Rossdale PD. Measurement of serum amyloid A in the neonatal foal using a latex agglutination immunoturbidimetric assay: determina-

tion of the normal range, variation with age and response to disease. Equine Veterinary Journal 2001; 33: 599-603.

[51] Hirvonen J., Pyörälä S. Acute phase response in dairy cows with surgically-treated abdominal disorders. The Veterinary Journal 1998; 155: 53-61.

[52] Gentry PA. Acute phase proteins. In: Loeb WF., Quimby FW. (eds.). Clinical chemistry of laboratory animals. Philadelphia: Taylor & Francis; 1999. p336-398.

[53] Thomas JS. Overview of plasma proteins. In: Feldman BF., Zinkl JG., Jain NC. (eds.). Schalm's Veterinary Hematology. Philadelphia: Lippincott Williams & Wilkins; 2000. p891-898.

[54] Rubel C., Fernandez GC., Dran G., Bompadre MB., Isturiz MA., Palermo MS. Fibrinogen promotes neutrophil activation and delays apoptosis. Journal of Immunology 2001; 166: 2002-2010.

[55] Aldred AR., Schreiber G. The negative acute phase protein. In: Mackiewicz I., Kushner I., Baumann H. (Eds.). Acute phase proteins. Molecular biology, biochemistry, and clinical applications. Boca Raton, Florida: CRC Press; 1993. p21-37.

[56] Mackiewicz A. Acute phase proteins and transformed cells. International Review of Cytology 1997; 170: 225-300.

[57] Stokol T., Tarrant JM., Scarlett JM. Overestimation of canine albumin concentration with the bromcresol-green method in heparinized plasma samples. Veterinary Clinical Pathology 2001; 30: 170-178.

[58] Pepys MB., Hirschfield GM. C-reactive protein: a critical update. Journal of Clinical Investigation; 111: 1805-1812.

[59] Mold C., Rodriguez W., Rodic-Polic B., Du Clos TW. C-reactive protein mediates protection from lipopolysaccharide through interactions with Fc-gammaR. Journal of Immunology 2002; 169: 7019-7025.

[60] Eckersall PD., Conner JG., Harvie J. An immunoturbidimetric assay for canine C-reactive protein. Veterinary Research Communications 1991; 15: 17-24.

[61] Yamamoto S., Shida T., Miyadi S., Santsuka H., Fujise H., Mukawa K., Furukawa E., Nagae T., Naiki M. Changes in serum C-reactive protein levels in dogs with various disorders and surgical trauma. Veterinary Research Communications 1993; 17: 85-93.

[62] Fournier T., Najet Medjoubi N., Porquet D. Alpha-1-acid glycoprotein: review. Biochimica et Biophysica Acta 2000; 1482: 157-171.

[63] Israili ZH., Dayton PG. Human Alpha-1-Glycoprotein and its interactions with drugs. Drug Metabolites Revue 2001; 33: 161-235.

[64] Tamura K., Yatsu T., Itoh H., Motoi Y. Isolation, characterization and quantitative measurement of serum a1-acid glycoprotein in cattle. Japanese Journal of Veterinary Science 1989; 51: 987-994.

[65] Segales J., Pineiro C., Lampreave F., Nofrarias M., Mateu E., Calsamiglia M., Andres J., Morales M., Pineiro M., Domingo M. Haptoglobin and pig-major acute protein are increased in pigs with postweaning multisystemic wasting syndrome (PMWS). Veterinary Research 2004; 35: 275-282.

[66] Snowder GD., van Vleck LD., Cundiff LV., Bennett GL. Bovine respiratory disease in feedlot cattle: Environmental, genetic, and economic factors. Journal of Animal Science 2006; 84: 1999-2008.

[67] Gänheim C., Hultén C., Carlsson U., Kindahl H., Niskanen R., Persson Waller K. The acute phase response in calves experimentally infected with bovine viral dirrhoea virus and/or *Mannheimia haemolytica*. Veterinary Medicine B 2003; 50: 1-8.

[68] Sivula NJ., Ames TR., Marsh WE., Werdin RE. Descriptive epidemiology of morbidity and mortality in Minnesota dairy heifer calves. Preventive Veterinary Medicine 1996; 27 (3-4): 155-171.

[69] Conner JG., Eckersall PD., Wiseman A., Bain RK., Douglas TA. Acute phase response in calves following infection with *Pasteurella haemolytica, Ostertagia ostertagi* and endotoxin administration. Research in Veterinary Science 1989; 47 (2): 203-207.

[70] Horadagoda NU., Eckersall PD. Immediate response in TNF-α and acute phase protein concentrations to infection with *Pasteurella haemolytica* A1 in calves. Research in Veterinary Science 1994; 57 (1): 129-132.

[71] Angen Ø., Thomsen J., Larsen LE., Larsen J., Kokotovic B., Heegaard PMH., Enemark JMD. Respiratory disease in calves: Microbiological investigations on trans-tracheally aspirated bronchoalveolar fluid and acute phase protein response. Veterinary Microbiology 2009; 137: 165-171.

[72] Tóthová Cs., Nagy O., Seidel H., Kováč G. The effect of chronic respiratory diseases on acute phase proteins and selected blood parameters of protein metabolism in calves. Berliner und Münchener Tierärztliche Wochenschrift 2010; 123 (7/8): 307-313.

[73] Dowling A., Hodgson JC., Schock A., Donachie W., Eckersall PD., McKendrick IJ. Experimental induction of pneumonic pasteurellosis in calves by intratracheal infection with *Pasteurella multocida* biotype A:3. Research in Veterinary Science 2002; 73: 37-44.

[74] Grell NS., Tjørnehøj K., Larsen LE., Heegaard PMH. Marked induction of IL-6, haptoglobin and INF-γ following experimental BRSV infection in young calves. Veterinary Immunology and Immunopathology 2005; 103 (3-4): 235-245.

[75] Nikunen S., Härtel H., Orro T., Neuvonen E., Tanskanen R., Kivelä S-L., Sankari S., Aho P., Pyörälä S., Saloniemi H., Soveri T. Association of bovine respiratory disease

with clinical status and acute phase proteins in calves. Comparative Immunology, Microbiology & Infectious Diseases 2007; 30: 143-151.

[76] Svensson C., Liberg P., Hultgren J. Evaluating the efficacy of serum haptoglobin concentration as indicator of respiratory-tract disease in dairy calves. The Veterinary Journal 2007; 174 (2): 288-294.

[77] Carter JN., Meredith GL., Montelongo M., Gill DR., Krehbiel CR., Payton ME., Confer AW. Relationship of vitamin E supplementation and antimicrobial treatment with acute-phase protein responses in cattle affected by naturally acquired respiratory tract disease. American Journal of Veterinary Research 2002; 63: 1111-1117.

[78] Berry BA., Confer AW., Krehbiel CR., Gill DR., Smith RA., Montelongo M. Effects of dietary energy and starch concentrations for newly received feedlot calves: II. Acute-phase protein response. Journal of Animal Science 2004; 82: 845–850.

[79] Humblet M-F., Coghe J., Lekeux P., Godeau J-M. Acute phase proteins assessment for an early selection of treatments in growing calves suffering from bronchopneumonia under field conditions. Research in Veterinary Science 2004; 77: 41-47.

[80] Jawor P., Stefaniak T. Acute phase proteins in treatment of calves with respiratory tract inflammation. Folia Universitatis Agriculturae Stetinensis, Zootechnica 2006; 48 (250): 51-56.

[81] Skinner JG., Brown RAL., Roberts L. Bovine haptoglobin response in clinically defined field conditions. Veterinary Record 1991; 128: 147–149.

[82] Svensson C., Lundborg K., Emanuelson U., Olsson SO. Morbidity in Swedish dairy calves from birth to 90 days of age and individual calf-level risk factors for infectious diseases. Preventive Veterinary Medicine 2003; 58 (3/4): 179-197.

[83] Piercy DWT. Acute phase responses to experimental salmonellosis in calves and colibacillosis in chicken: serum iron and caeruloplasmin. Journal of Comparative Pathology 1979; 89 (3): 309-319.

[84] Deignan T., Alwan A., Kelly J., McNair J., Warrens T., O'Farrelli C. Serum haptoglobin: an objective indicator of experimentally-induced *Salmonella* infection in calves. Research in Veterinary Science 2000; 69: 153-158.

[85] Jawor P. Determination of haptoglobin and fibrinogen during monitoring herd health and selected inflammatory states in cattle. PhD thesis. Wroclaw University of Environmental and Life Sciences; 2007.

[86] Tóthová Cs., Nagy O., Seidel H., Kováč G. Acute phase proteins in relation to various inflammatory diseases of calves. Comparative Clinical Pathology 2011, DOI 10.1007/s00580-011-1224-5.

[87] Muller-Doblies D., Arquint A., Schaller P., Heegaard PMH., Hilbe M., Albini S., Abril C., Tobler K., Ehrensperger F., Peterhans E., Ackermann M., Metzler A. Innate immune responses of calves during transient infection with a noncytopathic strain of

bovine viral diarrhoea virus. Clinical and Diagnostic Laboratory Immunology 2004; 11: 302-312.

[88] Werling D., Sutter F., Arnold M., Kun G., Tooten PC., Gruys E., Kreuzer M., Langhans W. Characterisation of the acute phase response of heifers to a prolonged low dose infusion of lipopolysaccharide. Research in Veterinary Science 1996; 61: 252-257.

[89] Gänheim C., Alenius S., Persson Waller K. Acute phase proteins as indicators of calf herd health. The Veterinary Journal 2007; 173: 645-651.

[90] Bradley AJ. Bovine mastitis: an evolving disease. The Veterinary Journal 2002; 164: 116-128.

[91] Sandholm M., Honkanen-Buzalski T., Kaartinen L., Pyörälä S. The bovine udder and mastitis. Jyväskylä, Finnland: Gummerus Kirjapaino Oy; 1995, p312.

[92] Gerardi G., Bernardini D., Elia CA., Ferrari V., Iob L., Segato S. Use of serum amyloid A and milk amyloid A in the diagnosis of subclinical mastitis in dairy cows. Journal of Dairy Research 2009; 76: 411-417.

[93] Conner JG., Eckersall PD., Doherty M., Douglas TA. Acute phase response and mastitis in the cow. Research in Veterinary Science 1986; 41 (1): 126-128.

[94] Hirvonen J., Pyörälä S., Jousimies-Somer H. Acute phase response in heifers with experimentally induced mastitis. Journal of Dairy Research 1996; 63 (3): 31-360.

[95] Hirvonen J., Eklund K., Teppo AM., Huszenicza G., Kulcsar M., Saloniemi H., Pyörälä S. Acute phase response in dairy cows with experimentally induced *Escherichia coli* mastitis. Acta Veterinaria Scandinavica 1999; 40: 35-46.

[96] Eckersall PD., Young FJ., McComb C., Hogarth CJ., Safi S., Weber A., McDonald T., Nolan AM., Fitzpatrick JL. Acute phase proteins in serum and milk from dairy cows with clinical mastitis. Veterinary Record 2001; 148: 35-41.

[97] Jacobsen S., Niewold TA., Kornalijnslijper E., Toussaint MJM., Gruys E. Kinetics of local and systemic isoforms of serum amyloid A in bovine mastitic milk. Veterinary Immunology and Immunopathology 2005; 104: 21-31.

[98] Pedersen LH., Aalbœk B., Røntved CM., Ingvartsen KL., Sørensen NS., Heegaard PMH., Jensen HE. Early pathogenesis and inflammatory response in experimental bovine mastitis due to *Streptococcus uberis*. Journal of Comparative Pathology 2003; 128: 156-164.

[99] Nielsen BH., Jacobsen S., Andersen PH., Niewold TA., Heegaard PMH. Acute phase protein concentrations in serum and milk from healthy cows, cows with clinical mastitis and cows with extramammary inflammatory conditions. The Veterinary Record 2004; 154: 361-365.

[100] Grönlund U., Sandgren CH., Persson Waller K. Haptoglobin and serum amyloid A in milk from dairy cows with chronic sub-clinical mastitis. Veterinary Research 2005; 36: 191-198.

[101] Kováč G., Tóthová Cs., Nagy O., Seidel H. Milk amyloid A and selected serum proteins in cows suffering from mastitis. Acta Veterinaria Brno 2011; 80: 3-9.

[102] Petersen HH., Gardner IA., Rossitto P., Larsen HD., Heegaard PMH. Accuracy of milk amyloid A (MAA) concentration and somatic cell count for diagnosing bovine mastitis. In: Proceedings of the 5th International Colloquium on Animal Acute Phase Proteins. 14-15 March 2005, Dublin, Ireland; 2005, p43-44.

[103] Nazifi S., Khoshvaghti A., Gheisari HR. Evaluation of serum and milk amyloid A in some inflammatory diseases of cattle. Iranian Journal of Veterinary Research 2008; 9: 222-226.

[104] Lippolis JD. Immunological signaling networks: integrating the body's immune response. Journal of Animal Sciences 2008; 86: E53-E63.

[105] Krakowski L., Zdzisińska B. Selected cytokines and acute phase proteins in heifers during the ovarian cycle course and in different pregnancy periods. Bulletin of the Veterinary Institue Pulawy 2007; 51: 31-36.

[106] Saini PK., Riaz M., Webert DW., Eckersall PD., Young CR., Stanker LH., Chakrabarti E., Judkins JC. Development of a simple enzyme immunoassay for blood haptoglobin concentration in cattle and its application in improving food safety. American Journal of Veterinary Research 1998; 59: 1101-1107.

[107] Gymnich S., Hiss S., Sauerwein H., Petersen B. Haptoglobin in sows at parturition. In: Proceedings of the Fourth European Colloquium on Acute Phase Proteins. Segovia, Spain; 2003, p136.

[108] Uchida E., Katoh N., Takahashi K. Appearance of haptoglobin in serum from cows at parturition. Journal of Veterinary Medical Science 1993; 55: 893-894.

[109] Ametaj B. A new understanding of the causes of fatty liver in dairy cows. Advances in Dairy Technology 2005; 17: 97-112.

[110] Tóthová Cs., Nagy O., Seidel H., Konvičná J., Farkašová Z., Kováč G. Acute phase proteins and variables of protein metabolism in dairy cows during the pre- and postpartal period. Acta Veterinaria Brno 2008; 77: 51-57.

[111] Chan JPW., Chang C-C., Hsu W-I., Liu W-B., Chen T-H. Association of increased serum acute-phase protein concentrations with reproductive performance in dairy cows with postpartum metritis. Veterinary Clinical Pathology 2010; 39 (1): 72-78.

[112] Alsemgeest SPM., Taverne MAM., Boosman R., van der Weyden BC., Gruys E. Peripartum acute-phase protein SAA concentration in plasma of cows and foetuses. American Journal of Veterinary Research 1993; 54: 164-167.

[113] Regassa F., Noakes DE. Acute phase protein response of ewes and the release of PGFM in relation to uterine involution and the presence of intrauterine bacteria. Veterinary Record 1999; 144: 502-506.

[114] Young CR., Eckersall PD., Saini PK., Stanker L. Validation of immunoassays for bovine haptoglobin. Veterinary Immunology and Immunopathology 1995; 49: 1-13.

[115] Alsemgeest SPM., vant Clooster GAE., van Miert ASJPAM., Huslkamp-Koch CK., Gruys E. Primary bovine hepatocytes in the study of cytokine induced acute-phase protein secretion *in vitro*. Veterinary Immunology and Immunopathology 1996; 53: 179-184.

[116] Chan JPW., Chu CC., Fung HP., Chuang ST., Lin YC., Chu RM., Lee SL. Serum haptoglobin concentration in cattle. Journal of Veterinary Medical Science 2004; 66: 43-46.

[117] Smith BI., Donovan GA., Risco CA., Young CR., Stanker LR. Serum haptoglobin concentrations in Holstein dairy cattle with toxic puerperal metritis. The Veterinary Record 1998; 142 (4): 83-85.

[118] Hirvonen J., Huszenicza G., Kulcsar M., Pyörälä S. Acute-phase response in dairy cows with acute postpartum metritis. Theriogenology 1999; 51 (6): 1071-1083.

[119] Huzzey JM., Duffield TF., LaBlanc SJ., Veira DM., Weary DM., Keyserlingk MAG. Haptoglobin as an early indicator of metritis. Journal of Dairy Science 2009; 92 (2): 621-625.

[120] Dubuc J., Duffield TF., Leslie KE., Walton JS., LeBlanc SJ. Risk factors for postpartum uterine diseases in dairy cows. Journal of Dairy Science 2010; 93 (12): 5764-5771.

[121] Mordak R. Usefulness of haptoglobin for monitoring the efficiency of therapy of fetal membrane retention in cows. Medycyna Weterynaryjna 2008; 64 (4A): 434-437.

[122] Warnick LD., Janssen D., Guard CL., Grohn YT. The effect of lameness on milk production in dairy cows. Journal of Dairy Science 2001; 84: 1988-1997.

[123] Stokka GL., Lechtenberg K., Edwards T., MacGregor S., Voss K., Griffin D., Grotelueschen DM., Smith RA., Perino LJ. Lameness in feedlot cattle. Veterinary Clinics of North America: Food Animal Practice 2001; 17: 189-207.

[124] Kujala M., Orro T., Soveri T. Serum acute phase proteins as a marker of inflammation in dairy cattle with hoof diseases. Veterinary Record 2010; 166: 240-241.

[125] Tóthová Cs., Nagy O., Seidel H., Paulíková I., Kováč G. The influence of hoof diseases on the concentrations of some acute phase proteins and other variables of the protein profile in heifers. Acta Veterinaria (Beograd) 2011; 61: 141-150.

[126] Laven RA., Livesey CT., May SA. Relationship between acute phase proteins and hoof horn haemorrhages in postpartum first-lactation heifers. Veterinary Record 2004; 154: 135-138.

[127] Smith BI., Kauffold J., Sherman L. Serum haptoglobin concentrations in dairy cattle with lameness due to claw disorders. The Veterinary Journal 2010; 186 (2): 162-165.

[128] Jawor P., Steiner S., Stefaniak T., Baumgartner W., Rzasa A. Determination of selected acute phase proteins during the treatment of limb diseases in dairy cows. Veterinary Medicine – Czech 2008; 53: 173-183.

[129] Jafarzadeh SR., Nowrouzian I., Khaki Z., Ghamsari SM., Adibhashemi F. The sensitivities and specificities of total plasma protein and plasma fibrinogen for the diagnosis of traumatic reticuloperitonitis in cattle. Preventive Veterinary Medicine 2004; 65: 1-7.

[130] McSherry BJ., Horney FD., deGroot JJ. Plasma fibrinogen levels in normal and sick cows. Canadian Journal of Comparative Medicine 1970; 34 (3): 191-197.

[131] Jawor P., Stefaniak T., Steiner S., Baumgartner W. Dynamics of selected acute phase proteins in surgical abomasal reposition in cows. Folia Veterinaria 2009; 53 (Suppl. LIII): 18-21.

[132] Nazifi S., Rezakhani A., Moaddeli A., Zarifi M., Gheisari HR. Study on diagnostic values of haptoglobin and serum amyloid A concentration in bovine heart diseases. Comparative Clinical Pathology 2009; 18: 47-51.

[133] Harding JC., Baarsch MJ., Murtaugh MP. Association of Tumor Necrosis Factor and acute phase reactant changes with post arrival disease in swine. Journal of Veterinary Medicine Series B 1997; 44: 405-413.

[134] Eurell TE., Bane DP., Hall WF., Schaeffer DJ. Srum haptoglobin concentration as an indicator of weight gain in pigs. Canadian Journal of Veterinary Research 1992; 56 : 6-9.

[135] Lauritzen B., Lykkesfeldt J., Skaanild MT., Angen Ø., Nielsen JP., Friis C. Putative biomarkers for evaluating antibiotic treatment of *Actinobacillus pleuropneumoniae* infection in pigs. Research in Veterinary Science 2003; 74: 271-277.

[136] Sorensen NS., Tegtmeier C., Andresen LO., Piňeiro M., Toussaint MJM., Campbell FM., Lampreave F., Heegaard PMH. The porcine acute phase protein response to acute clinical and subclinical experimental infection with *Streptococcus suis*. Veterinary Immunology and Immunopathology 2006; 113: 157-168.

[137] Francisco CJ., Shyrock TR., Bane DP., Unverzagt L. Serum haptoglobin concentration in growing swine after intranasal challenge with *Bordetella bronchiseptica* and toxigenic *Pasteurella multocida* type D. Canadian Journal of Veterinary Research 1996; 60: 222-227.

[138] Quereda JJ., Gómez S., Seva J., Ramis G., Cerón JJ., Muňoz A., Pallarés FJ. Acute phase proteins as a tool for differential diagnosis of wasting diseases in growing pigs. Veterinary Record 2012; 170 (21), doi: 10.1136/vr. 100005.

[139] Pallarés FJ., Martinez-Subiela S., Seva J., Ramis G., Fuentes P., Bernabé A., Muňoz A., Cerón, JJ. Relationship between serum acute phase protein concentrations and lesions in finishing pigs. The Veterinary Journal 2008; 177: 369-373.

[140] Chen HH., Lin JH., Fung HP., Ho LL., Yang PC., Lee WC., Lee YP., Chu RM. Serum acute phase proteins and swine health status. The Canadian Journal of Veterinary Research 2003; 67: 283-290.

Chapter 6

Molecular Aspects of Human Alpha-1 Acid Glycoprotein — Structure and Function

Kazuaki Taguchi, Koji Nishi,
Victor Tuan Giam Chuang, Toru Maruyama and
Masaki Otagiri

Additional information is available at the end of the chapter

http://dx.doi.org/10.5772/56101

1. Introduction

α_1-acid glycoprotein (AGP), also called *orosomucoid*, is an acute phase protein in blood. AGP is comprised of 183 amino acid residues and five N-linked oligosaccharides, with a molecular weight of approximately 44 kDa.[1-3] The five carbohydrate chains account for about 40% of the total mass and render AGP very soluble and confer acidic (pI~2.8-3.8) properties with a net negative charge at physiological pH.[1, 4] While AGP is mainly biosynthesized in the liver and secreted into the circulation,[5, 6] other organs including the heart, stomach and lungs have been reported to synthesize and secrete AGP as well.[1] The basal level of AGP is maintained at approximately 20 μmol/L in healthy individuals.

The biological role of AGP is not completely understood, albeit numerous *in vitro* and *in vivo* activities such as the inhibition of platelet aggregation, modulation of lymphocyte proliferation and drug transport, have been reported. [4, 7-10] AGP may be involved in various immunomodulatory or anti-inflammation events for the following two reasons. First, the expression of AGP is regulated by both cytokines (interleukin-1, interleukin-6 and tumor necrosis factor-α) and glucocorticoids, unlike other acute phase proteins including fibrinogen, ceruloplasmin and α_2-microglobulin, which only by interleukin-6.[11-14] The regulation of AGP production in human hepatocytes by glucagon, interleukin-8 and the interleukin-6 is thought to act via mitogen-activated protein kinase (MAPK) pathway. [15] Furthermore, endogenous and exogenous AGP was found to present at sites of inflammation in rats with inflammatory granuloma in a study using fluorescent labeled antibody to AGP or iodine125 labeled AGP. [16, 17] Secondly, it is well known that the plasma concentration of AGP is influenced by several factors. For example, stresses, inflammation, burns, infections and pregnancy etc. can increase AGP concentration from 2 - to 10 – fold.[18-20] In addition, drugs such as phenobarbital and rifampicin can also increase the concentration of AGP in plasma [21-24], *via* mechanisms that are independent of the inflammation pathway. [25-28]

Similar to plasma albumin, the binding and transportation of a range of endogenous and exogenous compounds is one of the major physiological functions of AGP.[29] Therefore, drug binding to AGP is important in terms of the correct understanding of pharmacokinetics of drugs, especially during acute phase conditions. We have been investigating the drug-binding specificity and pharmacokinetic properties of AGP using various biophysical and biochemical analytical methods such as spectrophotometry and protein engineering for the past twenty years. Furthermore, we recently succeeded in elucidating the first structure of the AGP (variant A) and its complex with drugs.[30]

In this chapter, a brief overview of the structures of the two AGP variants, characterization of the drug-binding, pharmacokinetic properties and the biological functions of AGP are discussed.

2. Variants of AGP

AGP exists as three main genetic variants with the genes located in tandem on chromosome 9.[31] The expression of AGP is under the control of three adjacent genes; AGP-A, which encodes the F1, F2 and S variants, whereas AGP-B and AGP-B′ encode the A variant.[32] All three genes are structurally similar to each other, the AGP B/B′ genes are identical whereas the AGP A gene contains 22 codon/base substitutions.[33] The precursor product of the AGP-A gene is a 201 amino acid polypeptide with a secretory N-terminal signal peptide of 18 residues. The F1 and S variants are distributed worldwide, but the F2 variant is limited to Europeans and West Asians.[34-36] The F1, F2 and S variants are generally collectively referred as F1*S, because they are encoded by two alleles of the ORM1 gene (AGP-A) differing in less than five amino acids (F1 has Gln-38/Val-174; F2 has Gln-38/Met-174 and S has Arg-38/Val-174). On the other hand, the A variant is coded by the ORM2 gene (AGP-B/B′) with approximately 20 amino acid substitutions. The F1*S and A variants differ in their amino acid sequences by approximately 20 residues out of a total of 183 residues (Figure 1).[37]

In most individuals, the molar ratio of the F1*S and A variants in blood typically ranges from 3:1 to 2:1.[36, 38] However, the relative proportions of the products of the AGP-A and AGP-B/B′ genes have been found to change during acute phase reactions.[39, 40] Vékey and co-workers reported that the molar ratio of the F1*S and A variants was in the vicinity of 8:1 in the plasma of lymphoma, melanoma and ovarian cancer patients.[41] This means that not only the total concentration of AGP but also the molar ratio of the F1*S and A variants may be altered under certain types of pathological conditions. As mentioned in the introduction, the binding and transportation of a range of endogenous and exogenous compounds is one of the major physiological roles of AGP.[29] Furthermore, the F1*S and A variants have different drug-binding selectivity (for details, see section "4", "drug-binding properties").[42] Therefore, an

http://dx.doi.org/10.5772/56101

	10	20	30
F1*S	QIPLCANLVP	VPITNATLDQ	ITGKWFYIAS
A	QIPLCANLVP	VPITNATLDR	ITGKWFYIAS
	40	50	60
	AFRNEEYNKS	VQEIQATFFY	FTPNKTEDTI
	AFRNEEYNKS	VQEIQATFFY	FTPNKTEDTI
	70	80	90
	FLREYQTRQD	QCIYNTTYLN	VQRENGTISR
	FLREYQTRQD	QCFYNSSYLN	VQRENGTVSR
	100	110	120
	YVGGQEHFAH	LLILRDTKTY	MLAFDVNDEK
	YEGGREHVAH	LLFLRDTKTL	MFGSYLDDEK
	130	140	150
	NWGLSVYADK	PETTKEQLGE	FYEALDCLRI
	NWGLSFYADK	PETTKEQLGE	FYEALDCLCI
	160	170	180
	PKSDVVYTDW	KKDKCEPLEK	QHEKERKQEE
	PRSDVMYTDW	KKDKCEPLEK	QHEKERKQEE
	183		
	GES		
	GES		

Figure 1. Amino acid sequence of the human AGP F1*S and A variants. Differences in the amino acid sequences of the two variants are shown in red letters.

increase in AGP concentration and a change in the ratio of the AGP (F1*S and A) variants would affect the pharmacokinetics and pharmacodynamics of drugs that are bound to AGP during inflammation and chronic disease.

3. Structure

3.1. Glycosylation

AGP has five N-linked glycans that make up more than 40% of the total mass of the molecule.[3] The N-glycosylation sites of AGP (Asn-15, -38, -54, -75, -85) can carry any one of the glycans shown in Figure 2 corresponding to different degrees of branching (bi-, tri-

and tetra-antennary).[1] These glycans are structurally heterogeneous due to the great diversity of the terminating sugars. As shown in Figure 2, sialic acid is one of the common terminating sugars, and can be linked to a galactose residue *via* either an α2-3 or α2-6 linkage. In addition, fucose is another known terminating sugar, which increases the expression of the four sialyl Lewis epitope (Lewis^X) in both acute and chronic inflammation conditions. [43-47] These different degrees of branching and terminating sugars cause the heterogeneity of AGP, at least 20 types of glycan structures in AGP have been reported. [48, 49] Halsall and coworkers investigated the distribution of oligosaccharides at the five glycosylation sites in distinct AGP variants using concanavalin A affinity-chromatography, reverse phase-high performance liquid chromatography (RP-HPLC) separation and off-line MALDI-Mass spectrometric analysis, and found that the percentage of the complex glycan type at each site in the three AGP variants was different.[50] In addition, using capillary liquid chromatography-electrospray mass spectrometry to characterize the N-linked glycosylation pattern of AGP, Imre *et al.* reported that (i) triantennary complex-type oligosaccharides predominate at site I (Asn-15) and II (Asn-38), (ii) tetra-antennary complex-type oligosaccharides predominate at sites III (Asn-54), IV (Asn-75) and V (Asn-85), (iii) sites IV and V also present a higher degree of branching and/or longer antennae.[51]

The glycosylation of AGP has been reported to change under various physiological and pathological states. [52] For example, a substantial increase in bi-antennary glycoforms as well as an increase in the degree of 3-fucosylation occurs in the early phase of an acute-phase reaction.[53] The AGP in cancer patients (lymphoma, ovarian tumor etc.) was found to have increased both sialylation and fucosylation, and different relative proportions of the total amounts of bi-, tri- and tetra-antennary sequences.[48, 54, 55] Furthermore, other pathological conditions like chronic inflammation, pregnancy, rheumatoid arthritis, alcoholic liver cirrhosis, sepsis are also known to cause changes in AGP glycosylation.[33, 56-60] Whether the changes in AGP glycosylation have any effect on the biological functions of AGP remains unknown. However, the presence of glycans has been reported to affect the conformational stability and post-translational modification of the folding process of glycoproteins, which include HIV-1 type-glycoprotein 123, quercetin 2, 3-dioxygenase, α_1-antitrypsin and prion protein.[61-64] Therefore, it is highly possible that the changes in AGP glycosylation that occur under various pathological conditions may serve to either protect the AGP protein from exogenous stress or facilitate various immunomodulatory or anti-inflammation events.

3.2. Protein

Highly heterogeneous carbohydrate chains of the AGP molecule makes it difficult to reveal the 3D-structure of AGP. For structural determination by X-ray crystallography, the glycans must be removed from AGP using enzymatic methods, but these procedures fail to completely remove all of the glycan structures, due to following reasons; (i) AGP must be denatured and the disulfide bonds must be reduced to allow the enzyme to digest all glycans. (ii) AGP that is enzymatically deglycosylated is much less soluble in water, thereby resulting in uneven digestion and may create a mixture of polymerized forms. Hence, structural data cannot be

http://dx.doi.org/10.5772/56101

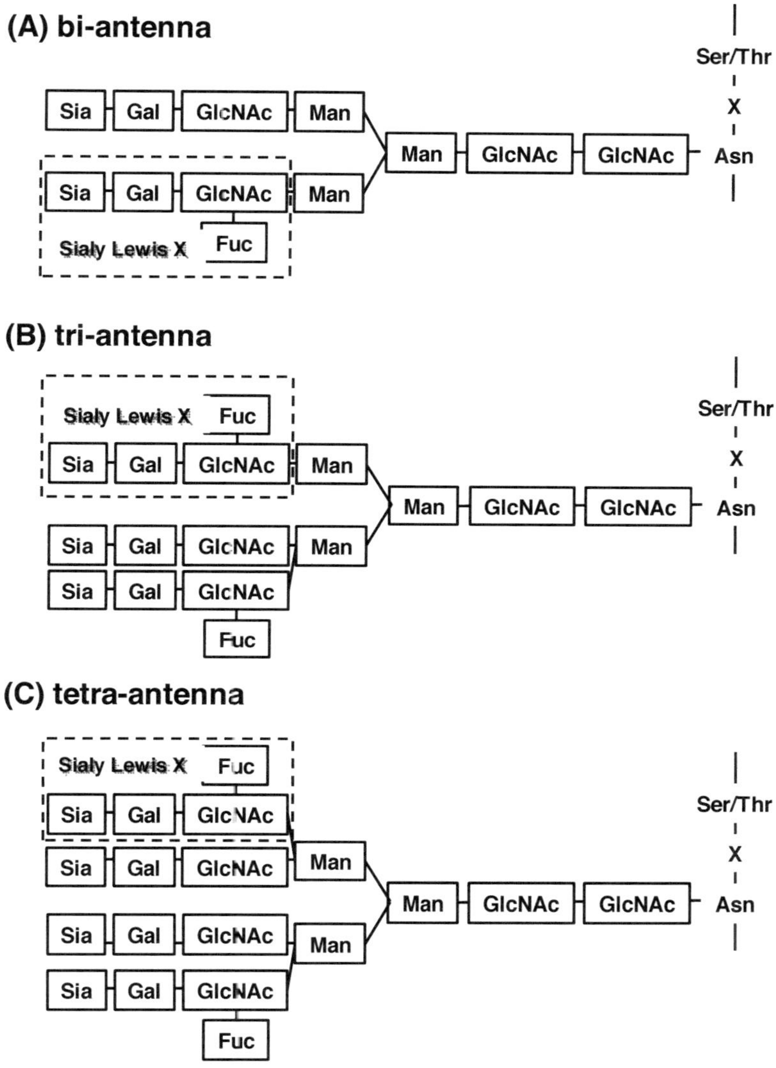

Figure 2. Di-, tri- and tetra-antennary N-linked complex glycans of human AGP. Dotted frame shows Sialy Lewis X. Man, mannose; GluNAC, N-acetylglucosamine; Fuc, fucose; Sia, sialic acid; Gal, galactose; Asn, asparagines; Ser, serine; Thr, threonine; X, any amino acid residue except proline

obtained from enzymatically deglycosylated AGP. In 2003, Kopecky *et al*. constructed a 3D-structure model of AGP using a combination of vibrational spectroscopy and molecular modeling, and concluded that folded AGP is a highly symmetrical all-beta protein that is dominated by a single eight-stranded antiparallel beta-sheet.[65] In addition, investigations using circular dichroism (CD) spectra and molecular modeling techniques suggest that AGP has an inherent tendency to form an α-helical structure and that His-172 of AGP plays an important role in the formation of an α-helical structure.[66-69]

Skerra and co-workers recently reported the first high-resolution X-ray structure of the recombinant unglycosylated F1*S variant of human AGP expressed from *Escherichia coli* at a 1.8 Å resolution (Figure 3A). [70] In addition, we have also determined the crystal structure of a C149R mutant of the human AGP A variant, in which a surface-exposed Cys residue was replaced by an Arg residue (as found in F1*S variant), using expression systems in *Escherichia coli* at a resolution of 2.1 Å (Figure 3B).[30] Our findings showed that the F1*S variant has a typical lipocalin folding pattern comprised of an eight-stranded β-barrel, corresponding to residues 24–32, 45–54, 58–68, 71–82, 86–92, 95–103, 109–114, and 123–128, respectively. On the other hand, the A variant is composed of eight β-strands, corresponding to 23–32, 44–54, 59–68, 71–82, 87–92, 95–102, 109–114, and 123–128, respectively. In addition, the F1*S variant contains the characteristic α-helix comprises residues 135–148 that packs against the β-barrel, and the A variant has four α-helices, 1–4, corresponding to 15–21, 35–42, 135–147. These results suggest that the overall folding pattern of F1*S and A variants are the same. It is noteworthy that the binding pocket of the F1*S variant is wide and consists of three lobes (I–III),[70] while, in the A variant, lobes I and II are maintained, but not lobe III.[30] This difference indicates that the binding region of the human AGP A variant is narrower than that of the F1*S variant, a difference that may be a contributing factor to the variants distinctive ligand binding selectivity.

4. Drug-binding properties

AGP exists in a mixture of two or three genetic variants. Herve′ *et al.* developed a method for fractionating AGP variants, which permitted the binding of drugs to the A and F1*S variants to be investigated,[71] and showed 35 chemically diverse drugs selectively binding to each variant. [71-73] The A variant showed higher drug binding selectivity than the F1*S variant, even though their structural properties are almost identical under physiological conditions. [74] These findings indicate that the drug-binding selectivity of AGP is dependent on the selectivity of the A variant, and that the F1*S variant binds a wider range of drugs. The X-ray crystallographic structures of AGP A and F1*S variants have recently been reported by two different groups showed that the binding pocket of the F1*S variant consists of three lobes (I–III) whereas two lobes (I and II) are involved in the case of the A variant.[30, 70] This result supports the view that the binding selectivity of the A variant is higher than that of the F1*S variant reported by Herve′ *et al.*[71-73] The crystal structures of the human AGP A variant complexed with disopyramide and amitriptyline, which bind to the A variant with a high degree of selectivity, reported by Nishi *et al.* recently revealed conserved edge-face contacts between the two aromatic rings on the drugs and the aromatic side chains of Phe-112 and Phe-49.[30] In addition, Ser-114 in the A variant is involved in a water-mediated hydrogen bond with the amide group of disopyramide. It is noteworthy that the residue at position 112 and 114 in the F1*S variant is leucine and phenylalanine, respectively. Therefore, the differences in the amino acid residues between the A and F1*S variants of AGP at positions 112 and 114 appear to be crucial for the high selectivity of the A variant for disopyramide, amitriptyline, and other A variant-specific drugs that contain two aromatic rings with similar configurations.

http://dx.doi.org/10.5772/56101

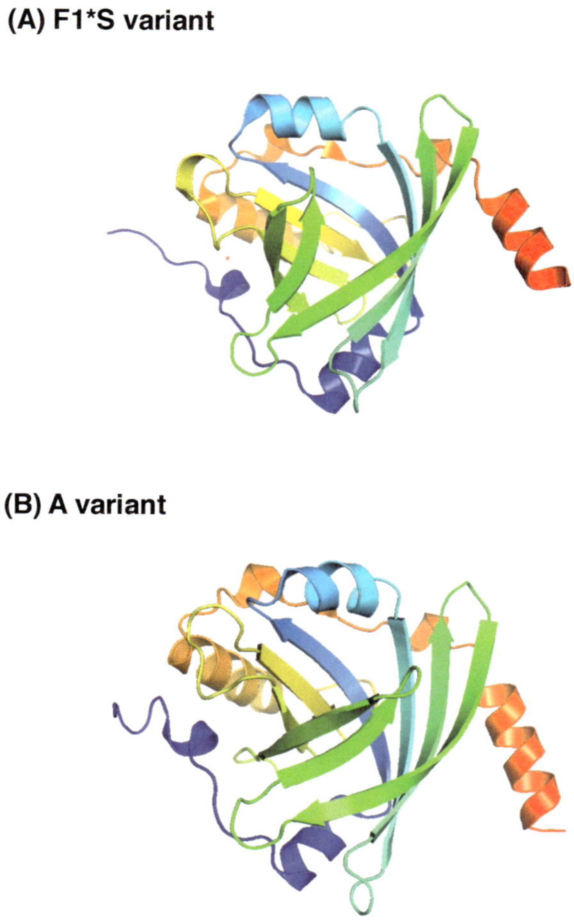

Figure 3. Figure 3 Crystal structures of the human AGP F1*S (A) and A variants (B) at a resolution of 1.8 Å and 2.1 Å, respectively. Both illustrations were produced with PyMol using the atomic coordinates from Protein Data Bank, 3KQ0 for (A) and 3APX for (B).

Molecular docking and modeling using the crystal structures of the A and F1*S variants are an alternate route to characterizing the drug-binding properties of AGP. Skerra and co-workers modeled the mode of binding of diazepam and progesterone to the F1*S variant, and predicted that (i) the polar diazepine ring of diazepam fits into the charged lobe II, resulting in the formation of two hydrogen bounds between the carbonyl oxygen to the side chains of Glu-64 and Gln-66, and that the two ring nitrogens were in contact with Arg-90 and Tyr-127, respectively. (ii) progesterone fitted nicely into lobe I and both Tyr-127 and Ser-40 was crucial for its binding.[70] Furthermore, Azad *et al*. characterized the binding properties of some polymyxin antibiotics (colistin, polymyxin B, polymyxin B_3, colistin methansulfonate, and colistin nonapeptide) with AGP using a combination of biophysical techniques, and developed a molecular model of the polymyxin B_3-AGP F1*S complex that showed the pivotal role of the N-terminal fatty acyl chain and the D-Phe6-L-Leu7 hydrophobic motif of polymyxin B_3 for binding to the cleft-like ligand binding cavity of the AGP F1*S variant.[75] In addition to these drugs, molecular docking models of imatinib, 6-mercaptopurine and thymoquinone, -AGP variants complex have also been developed.[76-78]

CD and fluorescence spectrometry is also a useful tool for examining the drug-binding sites of AGP. We found that electrostatic and hydrophobic forces have an important role in interactions between AGP and basic drugs.[79, 80] Furthermore, the results of fluorescent probe displacement experiments showed that basic drugs strongly displaced not only basic probes, but also acidic probes.[81] On the other hand, acidic probes were displaced by acidic drugs but had no effect on most of the basic probes. The results of the probe displacement study suggest that acidic drugs do not bind to an identical binding region as basic drugs, while acidic drugs do not share a binding region with basic drugs.

Photoaffinity labeling experiments and the use of chemically or genetically modified AGP can provide direct evidence for the specific amino acid residue that is involved in drug binding. The low distribution volumes of 7-hydroxystaurosporine (UCN-01), a protein kinase inhibitor anticancer drug,[82, 83] in patients was caused, in part, by its extraordinarily high affinity and specific binding ($Ka = 10^8\ M^{-1}$) to AGP.[84] Chemical modification of all His, Lys, Trp, and Tyr residues of AGP by reacting them with diethylpyrocarbonate, a phenyl isocyanate, 2-hydroxy-5-nitrobenzyl bromide, tetranitromethane, respectively, decreased the binding affinity of AGP to UCN-01.[83] In particular, Trp-modified AGP showed a significant decrease in binding. On the other hand, Zsila and Iwao used induced CD spectra and mutants of AGP to investigate its drug-binding sites, and reported that Trp25 is also involved in the binding of drugs to AGP.[85]

In addition, AGP mutants (W25A, W122A, and W160A)[86] photolabeled with [^{3}H]-UCN-01[87] revealed that only W160A showed a marked decrease in the extent of photoincorporation. These results strongly suggest that Trp-160 and Trp-25 play an essential role in the high affinity binding of UCN-01 to AGP. Furthermore, the displacement effects of propranolol, warfarin and progesterone on UCN-01-AGP binding were competitive in nature,[88] indicating that the UCN-01 binding site on AGP is partly overlapped with the binding site for basic drugs, acidic drugs, and steroid hormones.

Another investigation based on photoaffinity labeling experiments with [^{3}H]-flunitrazepam, also reported that [^{3}H]-flunitrazepam photolabeled an amino acid residue within the sequence of Tyr91-Arg105.[89] In addition, Kopecky *et al.*, using Raman difference spectroscopy, reported that Trp-122 is possibly involved in the binding of progesterone.[65] Furthermore, Halsall *et al.* reported that the modification of His-97 with diethylpyrocarbonate was inhibited in the presence of drugs that bind to AGP.[90] This finding suggests that, in addition to Trp-122, His-97 also participates in the binding of drugs. Based on the inconsistent results obtained from above mentioned studies, the binding sites do not appear to be completely separated, but overlap significantly and are influenced by one another, and that AGP has a wide drug-binding site that is common for basic, acidic and neutral drugs.

The unexpectedly high plasma concentrations of UCN-01 after intravascular administration in a clinical study in relation to preclinical studies (mice, rats, dogs) were found to be due to the high-affinity binding of UCN-01 to human AGP.[84] Investigation of species differences in the drug-binding properties of AGP is one of the important issues for the extrapolation of drug-protein interactions from animals to humans. We previously reported that both dog and bovine AGPs contain a basic ligand binding site and a steroid hormone binding site, which significantly overlaps and affects each other, but do not contain an acid ligand binding site.[91] On the other hand, the ligand binding site on human AGP consists of at least three partially overlapping subsites: a basic ligand binding site, an acidic ligand binding site and a steroid hormone binding site. Zsila *et al.* reported that chicken AGP is able to bind a broad spectrum of ligands, indicating the existence of a broad common drug binding site.[92]

Drugs bound to AGP have been proposed to be incorporated into cells of organs and tissues *via* membrane interactions.[93] The interaction of AGP with the membrane induces a structural change in AGP, followed by the release of the bound drug. We recently reported on the interactions of AGP with a model membrane using reverse micelles and liposomes.[68, 69] In the interaction with liposomes, AGP was found to bind to the surface of a membrane *via* electrostatic interaction. This interaction induced a structural change in AGP, which results in a decrease in its drug-binding capacity. An interesting finding was that AGP underwent a structural change to an α-helical form from a β-sheet form. We also found that the decrease in drug-binding capacity caused by the interaction with the membrane was dependent on the α-helix content of the AGP. These findings strongly suggest the existence of the AGP-mediated transport of drugs (Figure 4). It is important, in the future, to reveal how much this system contributes to overall drug transport into tissue.

5. Disposition

AGP is mainly biosynthesized in the liver and secreted into the blood circulation.[5, 6] In addition to the liver, other organs including the heart, stomach and lungs etc. are also able to synthesize and secrete AGP.[1] However, the disposition of endogenous AGP after being secreted into the circulation is not fully understood. In 1961, Weisman *et al.* performed the first pharmacokinetic study of AGP by administering ^{131}I-labelled human AGP to convalescent patients, and reported that the half-life of AGP in humans was approximately 5 days.[94] Bree *et al.* also administered ^{125}I-labelled human AGP (8.5 to 10 mg/patients) to seven male patients who were admitted in the intensive care unit due to brain injuries, and reported the half-life of AGP in humans (average half-life; 65 hour, range; 36.3-95.3 hour) was shorter than that observed by Weisman *et al.*.[95] In addition, they found that 60% of the administered AGP was located within the central compartment while the remaining 40% was present in the extravascular space like albumin.[96] These data indicated that the half-life of AGP is at least 2-3 days.

Keyler *et al.* studied the pharmacokinetics of high-doses of human AGP in rats and concluded that AGP could be safely cleared from the body even though the maximum serum AGP concentration after infusion was more than twenty times the normal value.[97] Pharmacoki-

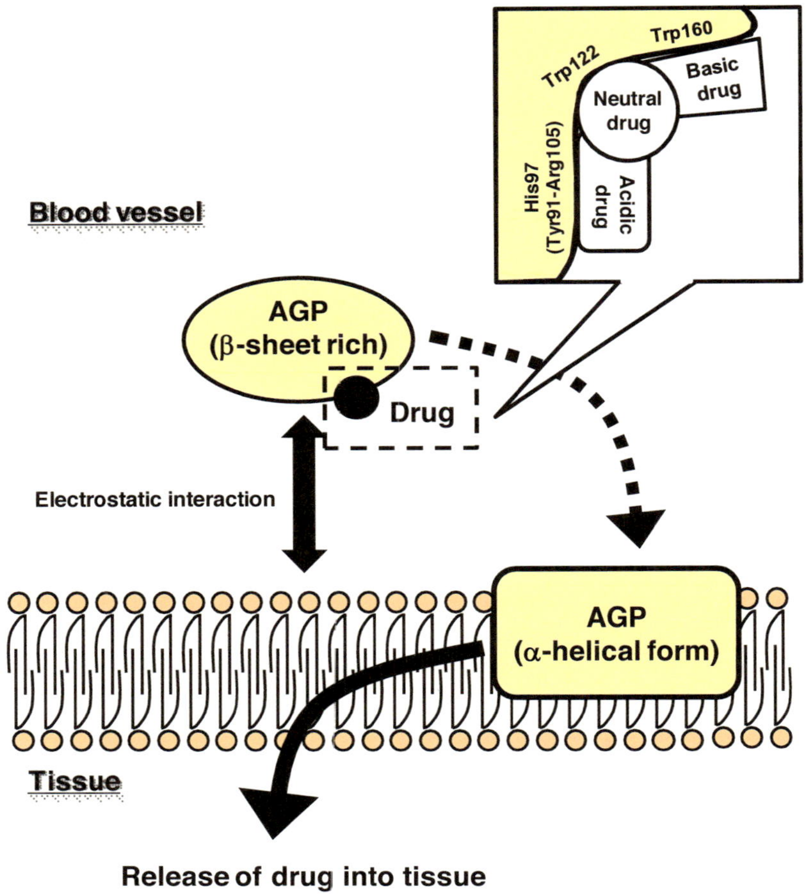

Figure 4. Proposed mechanism of AGP-mediated drug transport and drug-binding region of AGP. (modified from reference 29)

netic studies using mice and rabbits demonstrated that AGP was mainly distributed in the liver.[98, 99] We also clarified that AGP was mainly incorporated into liver parenchymal cells *via* a receptor-mediated pathway, and the hemoglobin β-chain located on liver plasma membranes contributes to the intracellular uptake of AGP.[100, 101] These data suggest that AGP is finally taken up by liver parenchymal cells *via* the hemoglobin β-chain and is then degraded or eliminated from the body.

The glycans of AGP are known to be largely responsible for the pharmacokinetic properties of the molecule, especially the elimination of AGP. The presence of glycans has been found to contribute in preventing accelerated clearance by glomerular filtration in the kidney, because AGP is a relatively small protein of approximately 44 kDa. In order to clarify the role of glycans in the renal elimination of AGP, we prepared a recombinant glycan-deficient AGP by mutating the five Asn residues to Asp residues using a Pichia expression system and studied the pharmacokinetics of this recombinant glycan-deficient AGP in mice.[101] The glycan-deficient AGP was eliminated from the blood circulation very rapidly, due to filtration in the kidney. In addition, McCurdy *et al.* also obtained similar results using glycan-deficient AGP in rabbits.[99]

An asialoglycoprotein receptor has been reported to be associated with the incorporation of AGP into liver tissue.[102] Regoeczi *et al.* studied the pharmacokinetics of asialo-AGP in chickens and rabbits, and suggested the possibility of the presence of a naturally occurring terminal catabolic point of AGP that was related to hepatic uptake *via* a hepatic plasma membrane receptor (an asialoglycoprotein receptor).[103] On the contrary, Ikeda *et al.* reported that the pharmacokinetics of AGP did not change in mice that lacked the asialoglycoprotein receptor compared to wild type mice.[104] In addition, the presence of a sialidase, which digests sialic acid from glycans, has identified in lysosomes [105, 106], cytoplasm [107, 108] and the plasma membrane [107, 109], but not in blood. These findings suggest that receptors other than the asialoglycoprotein receptor are involved in the incorporation of AGP into tissues. We investigated the pharmacokinetics of asialo-AGP (sialic acids removed), and agalacto-AGP (both sialic acids and galactose removed) in mice.[98] Whilst the elimination of ^{111}In labeled-AGP, -asialo-AGP and -agalacto-AGP from the circulation was suppressed by excess unlabeled AGP, asialo-AGP and agalacto-AGP, respectively, interestingly, agalacto-AGP but not asialo-AGP competed with AGP in uptake by the liver, while agalacto-AGP competed with asialo-AGP in uptake by the liver. In addition, the results from a mice study indicated that systemic hyaluronidase treatment decreased the initial clearance of AGP and that AGP administration reduced the binding of hyaluromic acid binding protein to the vessel wall of liver sinusoids. [99] These results suggest that AGP, including N-linked glycans, interact with hyaluronan or hyaluronidase-sensitive component of the vessel wall which influence the transendothelial passage of AGP. Based on these results, a new hepatic elimination pathway involving at least two types of receptors, namely an asialoglycoprotein receptor and another yet to be identified receptor, for AGP was proposed (Figure 5). This unidentified receptor is shared with AGP, and AGP is directly taken up by the liver through such a receptor and not *via* an asialoglycoprotein receptor.

The oligosaccharide chains of AGP have different degrees of branching (bi-, tri- and tetra-antennary) that is influenced by the physiological conditions. The pharmacokinetics of AGP, in turn, is also affected by the proportion of the bi-antennary glycans. Parivar *et al.* performed the disposition of concanavalin A (Con A)-non-reactive, which contains only one bi-antennary chains, and Con A-reactive human AGP, which contains two or more bi-antennary chains, in normal male rats and acute phase response-activated rats induced by treatment with ethynyloestradiol.[110] The clearance of both Con A-non-reactive and Con A-reactive human AGP was significantly increased in the acute phase response-activated rats compared to normal rats. The clearance of Con A-non-reactive human AGP was marginally higher than Con A-reactive human AGP in the acute phase response-activated rats, but no difference was found in the normal rats. These results indicate that the degree of branching of the glycans alters the disposition of AGP.

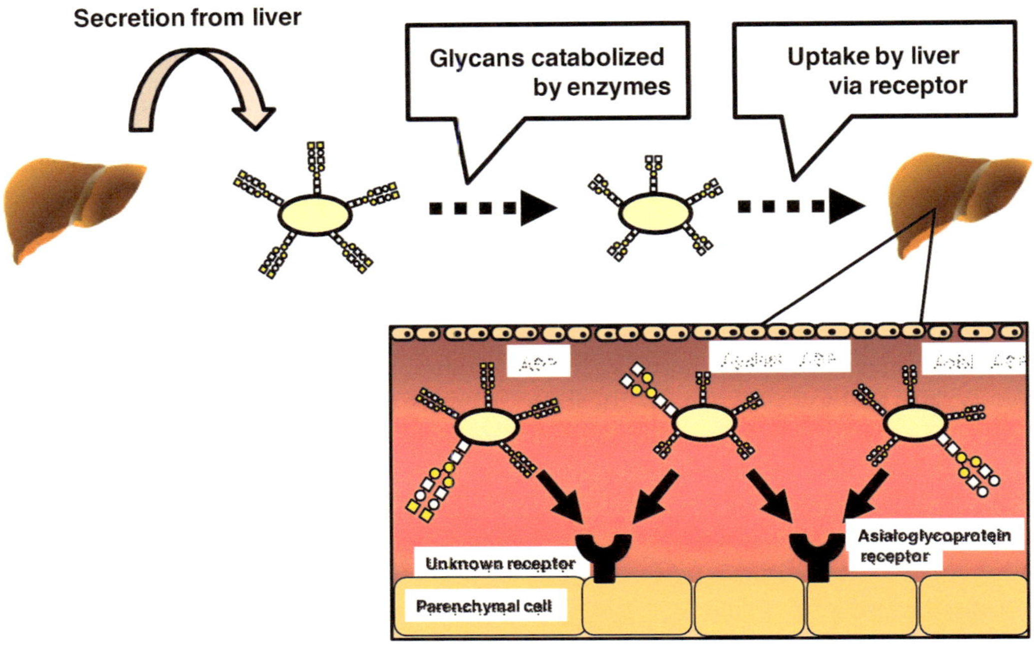

Figure 5. Proposed model of glycan dependent elimination pathway via transporter of AGP. yellow circle, mannose; open square, N-acetylglucosamine; yellow square, sialic acid; open circle, galactose

6. Biological functions

The several fold increase of AGP concentration in the circulation during an acute phase response could influence the biological functions of the molecule in humans. [111] Although the detailed biological functions of AGP has not been elucidated completely, the major physiological roles of AGP reported so far involve the binding and transport of a range of drugs and immunomodulating effects. These physiological roles of AGP have been reviewed in section "4" and elsewhere.[1, 4] Thus, the scope of this section is limited to some interesting observations for other roles.

Van Molle *et al*. found that bovine AGP with or without glycan chains inhibits the apoptosis of hepatocytes induced by TNF/galactosamine and TNF/actinomycin D in mice *via* suppressing the activation of caspase 3 and 7, which is a key factor in inducing apoptosis.[112, 113] On the contrary, Kagaya *et al*. reported that AGP inhibited the cell death of rat primary hepatocytes that had been treated with a chemical toxin (bromobenzene), and the hepatoprotective effect of AGP was lost when the sialic acid groups at the N-glycan chain terminal of AGP were removed.[114] In addition, Karande and co-workers demonstrated the importance of sialylation and glycan size in the manifestation of Glycodelin A for its induced apoptosis due to accessibility to the apoptogenic region.[115, 116] These results indicate that AGP potentially possesses anti-apoptosis or cytoprotective effects for hepatocytes which depends on both the presence/absence of glycans and the type of terminal sugar. Moreover, Buurman and co-workers demonstrated that human AGP decreases ischemia/reperfusion-induced damage to kidney tissue by suppressing apoptosis, the expression of TNF-α and neutrophil influx.[117, 118] They also found that AGP inhibited the activation of the complement system in the process, and that this protective effect was not associated with the fucosylation of the glycans of AGP. These findings indicate that AGP can be used as a potential new therapeutic intervention in the treatment of acute hepatic and renal failure, as seen after the transplantation of ischemically injured liver and kidneys.

AGP has also been reported to have a protective effect against sepsis from gram-negative infections.[119] Moore *et al*. showed that AGP interacts with the bacterial lipopolysaccharide (LPS), which is an initiator of the acute inflammatory response associated with septic shock, resulting in the formation of an AGP-LPS complex. This complexation by AGP neutralized the toxicity of LPS and enhanced the clearance of LPS from the body.[120] In addition, Hochepied *et al*. demonstrated that AGP was effective against a lethal infection by *Klebsiella pneumonia* and *Bacillus anthracis*.[119, 121] These results suggested that the increased AGP expression under conditions of an infection facilitates LPS elimination, resulting in a protective effect against endotoxin shock derived from the infection.

The effects of AGP on erythrocyte membranes have also been reported.[122-124] Maeda *et al*. showed that human AGP is bound to the surface of erythrocytes, which facilitated the passage of erythrocytes throughout artificial membrane filters with various pore diameters under positive pressure, and a pronounced protecting effect against hemolysis during the filtration was also observed.[122, 123] Furthermore, We demonstrated that human, dog and bovine AGPs are able to stabilize the erythrocyte membrane by binding to the surface of the erythrocyte.[124] At physiological concentrations, AGP protects erythrocytes from H_2O_2 due to its antioxidant activity.[124, 125] According to these reports, an increase in the AGP content in serum above the normal value found under pathological conditions facilitates the passage of erythrocytes through capillaries, stabilizes erythrocyte membranes and protects against oxidative stress, all of which are favorable properties for the microcirculation.

7. Conclusions

Since the initial discovery of AGP, numerous attempts have been made to study characteristics of the molecule, but the actual roles of AGP are yet to be fully understood. Recent advances in scientific technologies such as recombinant protein engineering provide novel and sophisticated tools to further elucidating the molecular and functional aspects of AGP. Among the recent findings, high-resolution X-ray structural data for recombinant the unglycosylated F1*S and A variants of human AGP would greatly promote the development of AGP research. In the near future, it is expected that AGP, like albumin, fibrinogen and immunoglobulin, will be developed for use in a variety of clinical situations.

Author details

Kazuaki Taguchi[1,5], Koji Nishi[1,2], Victor Tuan Giam Chuang[3], Toru Maruyama[1,4] and Masaki Otagiri[1,5,6*]

*Address all correspondence to: otagirim@ph.sojo-u.ac.jp

1 Department of Biopharmaceutics, Graduate School of Pharmaceutical Sciences, Kumamoto University, Kumamoto, Japan

2 Department of Clinical Pharmacokinetics and Pharmacodynamics, School of Medicine, Keio University, Shinjuku, Tokyo, Japan

3 School of Pharmacy, Faculty of Health Sciences, Curtin Health Innovation Research Institute, Curtin University, Perth, Western Australia, Australia

4 Center for Clinical Pharmaceutical Sciences, Kumamoto University, Kumamoto, Japan

5 Faculty of Pharmaceutical Sciences, Sojo University, Kumamoto, Japan

6 DDS Research Institute, Sojo University, Kumamoto, Japan

References

[1] Fournier T, Medjoubi NN, Porquet D. Alpha-1-acid glycoprotein. Biochim Biophys Acta 2000; 1482(1-2):157-171.

[2] Israili ZH, Dayton PG. Human alpha-1-glycoprotein and its interactions with drugs. Drug Metab Rev 2001;33(2):161-235.

[3] Schmid K, Nimerg RB, Kimura A, Yamaguchi H, Binette JP. The carbohydrate units of human plasma alpha1-acid glycoprotein. Biochim Biophys Acta 1977;492(2): 291-302.

[4] Hochepied T, Berger FG, Baumann H, Libert C. Alpha(1)-acid glycoprotein: an acute phase protein with inflammatory and immunomodulating properties. Cytokine Growth Factor Rev 2003;14(1):25-34.

[5] Athineos E, Kukral JC, Winzler RJ. Biosynthesis of Glycoproteins. Ii. The Site of Glucosamine Incorporation into Canine Plasma Alpha-1 Acid Glycoprotein. Arch Biochem Biophys 1964;106:338-342.

[6] Sarcione EJ. Sunthesis of alphal-acid glycoprotein by the isolated perfused rat liver. Arch Biochem Biophys 1963;100:516-519.

[7] Bories PN, Feger J, Benbernou N, Rouzeau JD, Agneray J, Durand G. Prevalence of tri- and tetraantennary glycans of human alpha 1-acid glycoprotein in release of macrophage inhibitor of interleukin-1 activity. Inflammation 1990;14(3):315-323.

[8] Gambacorti-Passerini C, Zucchetti M, Russo D, Frapolli R, Verga M, Bungaro S, et al. Alpha1 acid glycoprotein binds to imatinib (STI571) and substantially alters its pharmacokinetics in chronic myeloid leukemia patients. Clin Cancer Res 2003;9(2): 625-632.

[9] Pos O, Oostendorp RA, van der Stelt ME, Scheper RJ, Van Dijk W. Con A-nonreactive human alpha 1-acid glycoprotein (AGP) is more effective in modulation of lymphocyte proliferation than Con A-reactive AGP serum variants. Inflammation 1990;14(2):133-141.

[10] Williams JP, Weiser MR, Pechet TT, Kobzik L, Moore FD, Jr., Hechtman HB. alpha 1-Acid glycoprotein reduces local and remote injuries after intestinal ischemia in the rat. Am J Physiol 1997;273(5 Pt 1):G1031-1035.

[11] Baumann H, Prowse KR, Marinkovic S, Won KA, Jahreis GP. Stimulation of hepatic acute phase response by cytokines and glucocorticoids. Ann N Y Acad Sci 1989;557:280-295.

[12] Kulkarni AB, Reinke R, Feigelson P. Acute phase mediators and glucocorticoids elevate alpha 1-acid glycoprotein gene transcription. J Biol Chem 1985;260(29): 15386-15389.

[13] Kuribayashi T, Tomizawa M, Seita T, Tagata K, Yamamoto S. Relationship between production of acute-phase proteins and strength of inflammatory stimulation in rats. Lab Anim 2011;45(3):215-218.

[14] Stadnyk A, Gauldie J. The acute phase protein response during parasitic infection. Immunol Today 1991;12(3):A7-12.

[15] Wigmore SJ, Fearon KC, Maingay JP, Lai PB, Ross JA. Interleukin-8 can mediate acute-phase protein production by isolated human hepatocytes. Am J Physiol 1997;273(4 Pt 1):E720-726.

[16] Jamieson JC, Turchen B, Huebner E. Evidence for the presence of rat alpha 1-acid glycoprotein in granuloma tissue: a fluorescence microscopy study. Can J Zool 1980;58(9):1513-1517.

[17] Shibata K, Okubo H, Ishibashi H, Tsuda-Kawamura K, Yanase T. Rat alpha 1-acid glycoprotein: uptake by inflammatory and tumour tissues. Br J Exp Pathol 1978;59(6): 601-608.

[18] Cheresh DA, Haynes DH, Distasio JA. Interaction of an acute phase reactant, alpha 1-acid glycoprotein (orosomucoid), with the lymphoid cell surface: a model for nonspecific immune suppression. Immunology 1984;51(3):541-548.

[19] Fey GH, Fuller GM. Regulation of acute phase gene expression by inflammatory mediators. Mol Biol Med 1987;4(6):323-338.

[20] Stekleneva NI, Shevtsova AI, Brazaluk OZ, Kulinich AO. Expression and structural-functional alterations of α-1-acid glycoprotein at the pathological state. Biopolymers and Cell 2010;26(4):265-272.

[21] Abramson FP. Dose-response behavior of the induction of alpha 1-acid glycoprotein by phenobarbital in the dog. Drug Metab Dispos 1988;16(4):546-550.

[22] Abramson FP, Lutz MP. The kinetics of induction by rifampin of alpha 1-acid glycoprotein and antipyrine clearance in the dog. Drug Metab Dispos 1986;14(1):46-51.

[23] Chauvelot-Moachon L, Delers F, Pous C, Engler R, Tallet F, Giroud JP. Alpha-1-acid glycoprotein concentrations and protein binding of propranolol in Sprague-Dawley and Dark Agouti rat strains treated by phenobarbital. J Pharmacol Exp Ther 1988;244(3):1103-1108.

[24] Komori T, Kai H, Shimoishi K, Kabu K, Nonaka A, Maruyama T, et al. Up-regulation by clarithromycin of alpha(1)-acid glycoprotein expression in liver and primary cultured hepatocytes. Biochem Pharmacol 2001;62(10):1391-1397.

[25] Bertaux O, Fournier T, Chauvelot-Moachon L, Porquet D, Valencia R, Durand G. Modifications of hepatic alpha-1-acid glycoprotein and albumin gene expression in rats treated with phenobarbital. Eur J Biochem 1992;203(3):655-661.

[26] Fournier T, Mejdoubi N, Lapoumeroulie C, Hamelin J, Elion J, Durand G, et al. Transcriptional regulation of rat alpha 1-acid glycoprotein gene by phenobarbital. J Biol Chem 1994;269(44):27175-27178.

[27] Fournier T, Mejdoubi N, Monnet D, Durand G, Porquet D. Phenobarbital induction of alpha 1-acid glycoprotein in primary rat hepatocyte cultures. Hepatology 1994;20(6):1584-1588.

[28] Fournier T, Vranckx R, Mejdoubi N, Durand G, Porquet D. Induction of rat alpha-1-acid glycoprotein by phenobarbital is independent of a general acute-phase response. Biochem Pharmacol 1994;48(7):1531-1535.

[29] Otagiri M. A molecular functional study on the interactions of drugs with plasma proteins. Drug Metab Pharmacokinet 2005;20(5):309-323.

[30] Nishi K, Ono T, Nakamura T, Fukunaga N, Izumi M, Watanabe H, et al. Structural insights into differences in drug-binding selectivity between two forms of human alpha1-acid glycoprotein genetic variants, the A and F1*S forms. J Biol Chem 2011;286(16):14427-14434.

[31] Katori N, Sai K, Saito Y, Fukushima-Uesaka H, Kurose K, Yomota C, et al. Genetic variations of orosomucoid genes associated with serum alpha-1-acid glycoprotein

level and the pharmacokinetics of paclitaxel in Japanese cancer patients. J Pharm Sci 2011;100(10):4546-4559.

[32] Colombo S, Buclin T, Decosterd LA, Telenti A, Furrer H, Lee BL, et al. Orosomucoid (alpha1-acid glycoprotein) plasma concentration and genetic variants: effects on human immunodeficiency virus protease inhibitor clearance and cellular accumulation. Clin Pharmacol Ther 2006;80(4):307-318.

[33] Dente L, Ruther U, Tripodi M, Wagner EF, Cortese R. Expression of human alpha 1-acid glycoprotein genes in cultured cells and in transgenic mice. Genes Dev 1988;2(2): 259-266.

[34] Umetsu K, Yuasa I, Nishi K, Brinkmann B, Suzuki T. Orosomucoid (ORM) typing by isoelectric focusing: description of two new alleles in a German population and thermostability in bloodstains. Z Rechtsmed 1989;102(2-3):171-177.

[35] Yuasa I, Umetsu K, Suenaga K, Robinet-Levy M. Orosomucoid (ORM) typing by isoelectric focusing: evidence of two structural loci ORM1 and ORM2. Hum Genet 1986;74(2):160-161.

[36] Yuasa I, Weidinger S, Umetsu K, Suenaga K, Ishimoto G, Eap BC, et al. Orosomucoid system: 17 additional orosomucoid variants and proposal for a new nomenclature. Vox Sang 1993;64(1):47-55.

[37] Schmid K. Human plasma alpha 1-acid glycoprotein--biochemical properties, the amino acid sequence and the structure of the carbohydrate moiety, variants and polymorphism. Prog Clin Biol Res 1989;300:7-22.

[38] Eap CB, Baumann P. The genetic polymorphism of human alpha 1-acid glycoprotein. Prog Clin Biol Res 1989;300:111-125.

[39] Eap CB, Fischer JF, Baumann P. Variations in relative concentrations of variants of human alpha 1-acid glycoprotein after acute-phase conditions. Clin Chim Acta 1991;203(2-3):379-385.

[40] Hanada K, Yamanaka E, Yamamoto N, Minami H, Kawai S, Sasaki Y, et al. Effects of surgery and chronic disease states on the concentrations and phenotype distribution of alpha1-acid glycoprotein: studies in patients with breast cancer and patients with chronic inflammatory disease. Int J Clin Pharmacol Ther 2011;49(7):415-421.

[41] Budai L, Ozohanics O, Ludanyi K, Drahos L, Kremmer T, Krenyacz J, et al. Investigation of genetic variants of alpha-1 acid glycoprotein by ultra-performance liquid chromatography-mass spectrometry. Anal Bioanal Chem 2009;393(3):991-998.

[42] Fitos I, Visy J, Zsila F, Bikadi Z, Mady G, Simonyi M. Specific ligand binding on genetic variants of human alpha1-acid glycoprotein studied by circular dichroism spectroscopy. Biochem Pharmacol 2004;67(4):679-688.

[43] Brinkman-Van der Linden CM, Havenaar EC, Van Ommen CR, Van Kamp GJ, Gooren LJ, Van Dijk W. Oral estrogen treatment induces a decrease in expression of sialyl

Lewis x on alpha 1-acid glycoprotein in females and male-to-female transsexuals. Glycobiology 1996;6(4):407-412.

[44] Croce MV, Salice VC, Lacunza E, Segal-Eiras A. Alpha 1-acid glycoprotein (AGP): a possible carrier of sialyl lewis X (slewis X) antigen in colorectal carcinoma. Histol Histopathol 2005;20(1):91-97.

[45] Dage JL, Ackermann BL, Halsall HB. Site localization of sialyl Lewis(x) antigen on alpha1-acid glycoprotein by high performance liquid chromatography-electrospray mass spectrometry. Glycobiology 1998;8(8):755-760.

[46] De Graaf TW, Van der Stelt ME, Anbergen MG, van Dijk W. Inflammation-induced expression of sialyl Lewis X-containing glycan structures on alpha 1-acid glycoprotein (orosomucoid) in human sera. J Exp Med 1993;177(3):657-666.

[47] Ryden I, Pahlsson P, Lundblad A, Skogh T. Fucosylation of alpha1-acid glycoprotein (orosomucoid) compared with traditional biochemical markers of inflammation in recent onset rheumatoid arthritis. Clin Chim Acta 2002;317(1-2):221-229.

[48] Kremmer T, Szollosi E, Boldizsar M, Vincze B, Ludanyi K, Imre T, et al. Liquid chromatographic and mass spectrometric analysis of human serum acid alpha-1-glycoprotein. Biomed Chromatogr 2004;18(5):323-329.

[49] Kuster B, Hunter AP, Wheeler SF, Dwek RA, Harvey DJ. Structural determination of N-linked carbohydrates by matrix-assisted laser desorption/ionization-mass spectrometry following enzymatic release within sodium dodecyl sulphate-polyacrylamide electrophoresis gels: application to species-specific glycosylation of alpha1-acid glycoprotein. Electrophoresis 1998;19(11):1950-1959.

[50] Treuheit MJ, Costello CE, Halsall HB. Analysis of the five glycosylation sites of human alpha 1-acid glycoprotein. Biochem J 1992;283 (Pt 1):105-112.

[51] Imre T, Schlosser G, Pocsfalvi G, Siciliano R, Molnar-Szollosi E, Kremmer T, et al. Glycosylation site analysis of human alpha-1-acid glycoprotein (AGP) by capillary liquid chromatography-electrospray mass spectrometry. J Mass Spectrom 2005;40(11):1472-1483.

[52] Ceciliani F, Pocacqua V. The acute phase protein alpha1-acid glycoprotein: a model for altered glycosylation during diseases. Curr Protein Pept Sci 2007;8(1):91-108.

[53] van Dijk W, Havenaar EC, Brinkman-van der Linden EC. Alpha 1-acid glycoprotein (orosomucoid): pathophysiological changes in glycosylation in relation to its function. Glycoconj J 1995;12(3):227-233.

[54] Duche JC, Urien S, Simon N, Malaurie E, Monnet I, Barre J. Expression of the genetic variants of human alpha-1-acid glycoprotein in cancer. Clin Biochem 2000;33(3): 197-202.

[55] Hashimoto S, Asao T, Takahashi J, Yagihashi Y, Nishimura T, Saniabadi AR, et al. alpha1-acid glycoprotein fucosylation as a marker of carcinoma progression and prognosis. Cancer 2004;101(12):2825-2836.

[56] Biou D, Bauvy C, N'Guyen H, Codogno P, Durand G, Aubery M. Alterations of the glycan moiety of human alpha 1-acid glycoprotein in late-term pregnancy. Clin Chim Acta 1991;204(1-3):1-12.

[57] Biou D, Chanton P, Konan D, Seta N, N'Guyen H, Feger J, et al. Microheterogeneity of the carbohydrate moiety of human alpha 1-acid glycoprotein in two benign liver diseases: alcoholic cirrhosis and acute hepatitis. Clin Chim Acta 1989;186(1):59-66.

[58] Jezequel M, Seta NS, Corbic MM, Feger JM, Durand GM. Modifications of concanavalin A patterns of alpha 1-acid glycoprotein and alpha 2-HS glycoprotein in alcoholic liver disease. Clin Chim Acta 1988;176(1):49-57.

[59] Serbource-Goguel Seta N, Durand G, Corbic M, Agneray J, Fegar J. Alterations in relative proportions of microheterogenous forms of human alpha 1-acid glycoprotein in liver disease. J Hepatol 1986;2(2):245-252.

[60] Wieruszeski JM, Fournet B, Konan D, Biou D, Durand G. 400-MHz 1H-NMR spectroscopy of fucosylated tetrasialyl oligosaccharides isolated from normal and cirrhotic alpha 1-acid glycoprotein. FEBS Lett 1988;238(2):390-394.

[61] Fusetti F, Schroter KH, Steiner RA, van Noort PI, Pijning T, Rozeboom HJ, et al. Crystal structure of the copper-containing quercetin 2,3-dioxygenase from Aspergillus japonicus. Structure 2002;10(2):259-268.

[62] Kwon KS, Yu MH. Effect of glycosylation on the stability of alpha1-antitrypsin toward urea denaturation and thermal deactivation. Biochim Biophys Acta 1997;1335(3):265-272.

[63] Lehmann S, Harris DA. Blockade of glycosylation promotes acquisition of scrapie-like properties by the prion protein in cultured cells. J Biol Chem 1997;272(34): 21479-21487.

[64] Li Y, Luo L, Rasool N, Kang CY. Glycosylation is necessary for the correct folding of human immunodeficiency virus gp120 in CD4 binding. J Virol 1993;67(1):584-588.

[65] Kopecky V, Jr., Ettrich R, Hofbauerova K, Baumruk V. Structure of human alpha1-acid glycoprotein and its high-affinity binding site. Biochem Biophys Res Commun 2003;300(1):41-46.

[66] Aubert JP, Loucheux-Lefebvre MH. Conformational study of alpha1-acid glycoprotein. Arch Biochem Biophys 1976;175(2):400-409.

[67] Nishi K, Komine Y, Fukunaga N, Maruyama T, Suenaga A, Otagiri M. Involvement of disulfide bonds and histidine 172 in a unique beta-sheet to alpha-helix transition

of alpha 1-acid glycoprotein at the biomembrane interface. Proteins 2006;63(3): 611-620.

[68] Nishi K, Maruyama T, Halsall HB, Handa T, Otagiri M. Binding of alpha1-acid glycoprotein to membrane results in a unique structural change and ligand release. Biochemistry 2004;43(32):10513-10519.

[69] Nishi K, Sakai N, Komine Y, Maruyama T, Halsall HB, Otagiri M. Structural and drug-binding properties of alpha(1)-acid glycoprotein in reverse micelles. Biochim Biophys Acta 2002;1601(2):185-191.

[70] Schonfeld DL, Ravelli RB, Mueller U, Skerra A. The 1.8-A crystal structure of alpha1-acid glycoprotein (Orosomucoid) solved by UV RIP reveals the broad drug-binding activity of this human plasma lipocalin. J Mol Biol 2008;384(2):393-405.

[71] Herve F, Caron G, Duche JC, Gaillard P, Abd Rahman N, Tsantili-Kakoulidou A, et al. Ligand specificity of the genetic variants of human alpha1-acid glycoprotein: generation of a three-dimensional quantitative structure-activity relationship model for drug binding to the A variant. Mol Pharmacol 1998;54(1):129-138.

[72] Herve F, Duche JC, d'Athis P, Marche C, Barre J, Tillement JP. Binding of disopyramide, methadone, dipyridamole, chlorpromazine, lignocaine and progesterone to the two main genetic variants of human alpha 1-acid glycoprotein: evidence for drug-binding differences between the variants and for the presence of two separate drug-binding sites on alpha 1-acid glycoprotein. Pharmacogenetics 1996;6(5):403-415.

[73] Herve F, Gomas E, Duche JC, Tillement JP. Evidence for differences in the binding of drugs to the two main genetic variants of human alpha 1-acid glycoprotein. Br J Clin Pharmacol 1993;36(3):241-249.

[74] Kuroda Y, Matsumoto S, Shibukawa A, Nakagawa T. Capillary electrophoretic study on pH dependence of enantioselective disopyramide binding to genetic variants of human alpha1-acid glycoprotein. Analyst 2003;128(8):1023-1027.

[75] Azad MA, Huang JX, Cooper MA, Roberts KD, Thompson PE, Nation RL, et al. Structure-activity relationships for the binding of polymyxins with human alpha-1-acid glycoprotein. Biochem Pharmacol 2012;84(3):278-291.

[76] Fitos I, Simon A, Zsila F, Mady G, Bencsura A, Varga Z, et al. Characterization of binding mode of imatinib to human alpha1-acid glycoprotein. Int J Biol Macromol 2012;50(3):788-795.

[77] Lupidi G, Camaioni E, Khalife H, Avenali L, Damiani E, Tanfani F, et al. Characterization of thymoquinone binding to human alpha(1) -acid glycoprotein. J Pharm Sci 2012;101(7):2564-2573.

[78] Sochacka J, Pawelczak B. Characterization of 6-mercaptopurine binding site on human alpha1-acid glycoprotein (orosomucoid) using molecular docking. Acta Pol Pharm 2012;69(1):161-166.

[79] Miyoshi T, Sukimoto K, Otagiri M. Investigation of the interaction mode of phenothiazine neuroleptics with alpha 1-acid glycoprotein. J Pharm Pharmacol 1992;44(1): 28-33.

[80] Rahman MH, Miyoshi T, Sukimoto K, Takadate A, Otagiri M. Interaction mode of dicumarol and its derivatives with human serum albumin, alpha 1-acid glycoprotein and asialo alpha 1-acid glycoprotein. J Pharmacobiodyn 1992;15(1):7-16.

[81] Maruyama T, Otagiri M, Takadate A. Characterization of drug binding sites on alpha 1-acid glycoprotein. Chem Pharm Bull (Tokyo) 1990;38(6):1688-1691.

[82] Fuse E, Kuwabara T, Sparreboom A, Sausville EA, Figg WD. Review of UCN-01 development: a lesson in the importance of clinical pharmacology. J Clin Pharmacol 2005;45(4):394-403.

[83] Katsuki M, Chuang VT, Nishi K, Suenaga A, Otagiri M. Tryptophan residues play an important role in the extraordinarily high affinity binding interaction of UCN-01 to human alpha-1-acid glycoprotein. Pharm Res 2004;21(9):1648-1655.

[84] Fuse E, Tanii H, Kurata N, Kobayashi H, Shimada Y, Tamura T, et al. Unpredicted clinical pharmacology of UCN-01 caused by specific binding to human alpha1-acid glycoprotein. Cancer Res 1998;58(15):3248-3253.

[85] Zsila F, Iwao Y. The drug binding site of human alpha1-acid glycoprotein: insight from induced circular dichroism and electronic absorption spectra. Biochim Biophys Acta 2007;1770(5):797-809.

[86] Nishi K, Fukunaga N, Otagiri M. Construction of expression system for human alpha 1-acid glycoprotein in Pichia pastoris and evaluation of its drug-binding properties. Drug Metab Dispos 2004;32(10):1069-1074.

[87] Katsuki M, Chuang VT, Nishi K, Kawahara K, Nakayama H, Yamaotsu N, et al. Use of photoaffinity labeling and site-directed mutagenesis for identification of the key residue responsible for extraordinarily high affinity binding of UCN-01 in human alpha1-acid glycoprotein. J Biol Chem 2005;280(2):1384-1391.

[88] Kurata N, Matsushita S, Nishi K, Watanabe HH, Kobayashi S, Suenaga A, et al. Characterization of a binding site of UCN-01, a novel anticancer drug on alpha-acid glycoprotein. Biol Pharm Bull 2000;23(7):893-895.

[89] Chuang VT, Hijioka M, Katsuki M, Nishi K, Hara T, Kaneko K, et al. Characterization of benzodiazepine binding site on human alpha1-acid glycoprotein using flunitrazepam as a photolabeling agent. Biochim Biophys Acta 2005;1725(3):385-393.

[90] Halsall HB, Austin RC, Dage JL, Sun H, Schlueter KT. Structural aspects of alpha 1-acid glycoprotein and its interaction. Proc int Symp on Serum Albumin and Alpha 1-acid Glycoprotein, Tokyo Print, Kumamoto, Japan 2000:44-54.

[91] Matsumoto K, Sukimoto K, Nishi K, Maruyama T, Suenaga A, Otagiri M. Characterization of ligand binding sites on the alpha1-acid glycoprotein in humans, bovines and dogs. Drug Metab Pharmacokinet 2002;17(4):300-306.

[92] Zsila F, Matsunaga H, Bikadi Z, Haginaka J. Multiple ligand-binding properties of the lipocalin member chicken alpha1-acid glycoprotein studied by circular dichroism and electronic absorption spectroscopy: the essential role of the conserved tryptophan residue. Biochim Biophys Acta 2006;1760(8):1248-1273.

[93] Lin TH, Sawada Y, Sugiyama Y, Iga T, Hanano M. Effects of albumin and alpha 1-acid glycoprotein on the transport of imipramine and desipramine through the blood-brain barrier in rats. Chem Pharm Bull (Tokyo) 1987;35(1):294-301.

[94] Weisman S, Goldsmith B, Winzler R, Lepper MH. Turnover of plasma orosomucoid in man. J Lab Clin Med 1961;57:7-15.

[95] Bree F, Houin G, Barre J, Moretti JL, Wirquin V, Tillement JP. Pharmacokinetics of intravenously administered 125I-labelled human alpha 1-acid glycoprotein. Clin Pharmacokinet 1986;11(4):336-342.

[96] Berson SA, Yalow RS, Schreiber SS, Post J. Tracer experiments with I131 labeled human serum albumin: distribution and degradation studies. J Clin Invest 1953;32(8): 746-768.

[97] Keyler DE, Pentel PR, Haughey DB. Pharmacokinetics and toxicity of high-dose human alpha 1-acid glycoprotein infusion in the rat. J Pharm Sci 1987;76(2):101-104.

[98] Matsumoto K, Nishi K, Kikuchi M, Watanabe H, Nakajou K, Komori H, et al. Receptor-mediated uptake of human alpha1-acid glycoprotein into liver parenchymal cells in mice. Drug Metab Pharmacokinet 2010;25(1):101-107.

[99] McCurdy TR, Bhakta V, Eltringham-Smith LJ, Gataiance S, Fox-Robichaud AE, Sheffield WP. In vivo clearance of alpha-1 acid glycoprotein is influenced by the extent of its N-linked glycosylation and by its interaction with the vessel wall. J Biomed Biotechnol 2012; 292730.

[100] Komori H, Nishi K, Uehara N, Watanabe H, Shuto T, Suenaga A, et al. Characterization of hepatic cellular uptake of alpha1-acid glycoprotein (AGP), part 2: involvement of hemoglobin beta-chain on plasma membranes in the uptake of human AGP by liver parenchymal cells. J Pharm Sci 2012;101(4):1607-1615.

[101] Nishi K, Komori H, Kikuchi M, Uehara N, Fukunaga N, Matsumoto K, et al. Characterization of the hepatic cellular uptake of alpha(1) -acid glycoprotein (AGP), part 1: a peptide moiety of human AGP is recognized by the hemoglobin beta-chain on mouse liver parenchymal cells. J Pharm Sci 2012;101(4):1599-1606.

[102] Morell AG, Gregoriadis G, Scheinberg IH, Hickman J, Ashwell G. The role of sialic acid in determining the survival of glycoproteins in the circulation. J Biol Chem 1971;246(5):1461-1467.

[103] Regoeczi E, Hatton MW, Charlwood PA. Carbohydrate-mediated elimination of avian plasma glycoprotein in mammals. Nature 1975;254(5502):699-701.

[104] Ishibashi S, Hammer RE, Herz J. Asialoglycoprotein receptor deficiency in mice lacking the minor receptor subunit. J Biol Chem 1994;269(45):27803-27806.

[105] Milner CM, Smith SV, Carrillo MB, Taylor GL, Hollinshead M, Campbell RD. Identification of a sialidase encoded in the human major histocompatibility complex. J Biol Chem 1997;272(7):4549-4558.

[106] Pshezhetsky AV, Richard C, Michaud L, Igdoura S, Wang S, Elsliger MA, et al. Cloning, expression and chromosomal mapping of human lysosomal sialidase and characterization of mutations in sialidosis. Nat Genet 1997;15(3):316-320.

[107] Miyagi T, Wada T, Iwamatsu A, Hata K, Yoshikawa Y, Tokuyama S, et al. Molecular cloning and characterization of a plasma membrane-associated sialidase specific for gangliosides. J Biol Chem 1999;274(8):5004-5011.

[108] Monti E, Preti A, Rossi E, Ballabio A, Borsani G. Cloning and characterization of NEU2, a human gene homologous to rodent soluble sialidases. Genomics 1999;57(1): 137-143.

[109] Wada T, Yoshikawa Y, Tokuyama S, Kuwabara M, Akita H, Miyagi T. Cloning, expression, and chromosomal mapping of a human ganglioside sialidase. Biochem Biophys Res Commun 1999;261(1):21-27.

[110] Parivar K, Tolentino L, Taylor G, Oie S. Elimination of non-reactive and weakly reactive human alpha 1-acid glycoprotein after induction of the acute phase response in rats. J Pharm Pharmacol 1992;44(5):447-450.

[111] Kremer JM, Wilting J, Janssen LH. Drug binding to human alpha-1-acid glycoprotein in health and disease. Pharmacol Rev 1988;40(1):1-47.

[112] Van Molle W, Denecker G, Rodriguez I, Brouckaert P, Vandenabeele P, Libert C. Activation of caspases in lethal experimental hepatitis and prevention by acute phase proteins. J Immunol 1999;163(10):5235-5241.

[113] Van Molle W, Libert C, Fiers W, Brouckaert P. Alpha 1-acid glycoprotein and alpha 1-antitrypsin inhibit TNF-induced but not anti-Fas-induced apoptosis of hepatocytes in mice. J Immunol 1997;159(7):3555-3564.

[114] Kagaya N, Kamiyoshi A, Tagawa Y, Akamatsu S, Isoda K, Kawase M, et al. Suppression of cell death in primary rat hepatocytes by alpha1-acid glycoprotein. J Biosci Bioeng 2005;99(1):81-83.

[115] Jayachandran R, Radcliffe CM, Royle L, Harvey DJ, Dwek RA, Rudd PM, et al. Oligosaccharides modulate the apoptotic activity of glycodelin. Glycobiology 2006;16(11): 1052-1063.

[116] Mukhopadhyay D, SundarRaj S, Alok A, Karande AA. Glycodelin A, not glycodelin S, is apoptotically active. Relevance of sialic acid modification. J Biol Chem 2004;279(10):8577-8584.

[117] Daemen MA, Heemskerk VH, van't Veer C, Denecker G, Wolfs TG, Vandenabeele P, et al. Functional protection by acute phase proteins alpha(1)-acid glycoprotein and alpha(1)-antitrypsin against ischemia/reperfusion injury by preventing apoptosis and inflammation. Circulation 2000;102(12):1420-1426.

[118] de Vries B, Walter SJ, Wolfs TG, Hochepied T, Rabina J, Heeringa P, et al. Exogenous alpha-1-acid glycoprotein protects against renal ischemia-reperfusion injury by inhibition of inflammation and apoptosis. Transplantation 2004;78(8):1116-1124.

[119] Hochepied T, Van Molle W, Berger FG, Baumann H, Libert C. Involvement of the acute phase protein alpha 1-acid glycoprotein in nonspecific resistance to a lethal gram-negative infection. J Biol Chem 2000;275(20):14903-14909.

[120] Moore DF, Rosenfeld MR, Gribbon PM, Winlove CP, Tsai CM. Alpha-1-acid (AAG, orosomucoid) glycoprotein: interaction with bacterial lipopolysaccharide and protection from sepsis. Inflammation 1997;21(1):69-82.

[121] Shemyakin IG, Pukhalsky AL, Stepanshina VN, Shmarina GV, Aleshkin VA, Afanas'ev SS. Preventive and therapeutic effects of alpha-acid glycoprotein in mice infected with B. anthracis. Bull Exp Biol Med 2005;140(4):439-444.

[122] Maeda H, Morinaga T, Mori I, Nishi K. Further characterization of the effects of alpha-1-acid glycoprotein on the passage of human erythrocytes through micropores. Cell Struct Funct 1984;9(3):279-290.

[123] Maeda H, Nishi K, Mori I. Facilitating effects of alpha-1 acid glycoprotein on the passage of erythrocytes through the membrane-filter. Life Sci 1980;27(2):157-161.

[124] Matsumoto K, Nishi K, Tokutomi Y, Irie T, Suenaga A, Otagiri M. Effects of alpha 1-acid glycoprotein on erythrocyte deformability and membrane stabilization. Biol Pharm Bull 2003;26(1):123-126.

[125] Pukhal'skii AL, Shmarina GV, Kalashnikova EA, Shiyan SD, Kokarovtseva SN, Pukhal'skaya DA, et al. Effect of semisynthetic analog of alpha(1)-acid glycoprotein on immunomodulatory and antiinflammatory activity of natural glycoprotein. Bull Exp Biol Med 2000;129(5):480-483.

Chapter 7

Unique Assembly Structure of Human Haptoglobin Phenotypes 1-1, 2-1, and 2-2 and a Predominant Hp 1 Allele Hypothesis

Mikael Larsson, Tsai-Mu Cheng,
Cheng-Yu Chen and Simon J. T. Mao

Additional information is available at the end of the chapter

http://dx.doi.org/10.5772/56048

1. Introduction

Haptoglobin (Hp) is an acute phase protein present in the plasma of all mammals [1, 2]. One important function of Hp is its high binding affinity to hemoglobin (Hb) in forming the Hp-Hb complex that is metabolized through a receptor mediated process involving CD 163 of macrophages[3, 4]. This function is clinically relevant since Hb possesses a highly oxidative heme-group, producing reactive oxygen species when released from the red blood cells. On the contrary, Hp is a potent antioxidant which is stronger than the therapeutic agent probucol, which protects cells against oxidative stress [1, 5].

In humans there are two common alleles, *Hp 1* and *Hp 2*, corresponding to $\alpha1\beta$ and $\alpha2\beta$ polypeptide chains, respectively[3, 6]. All the phenotypes share the same β chain that is comprised of 245 amino-acid residues (Mw 40 kDa). As shown in Figure 1A, $\alpha1$ contains 83 amino-acid residues (Mw 9 kDa) and possesses two free –SH groups. The one at the –COOH terminus Cys-72 always crosslinks with a β chain to form a basic $\alpha\beta$ unit or ($\alpha1\beta$), and the other one at the NH2-terminus Cys-15 has to link with another ($\alpha1\beta$) unit resulting in a Hp dimer ($\alpha1\beta$)2 or Hp 1-1. In contrast, the $\alpha2$ chain contains the same residues as $\alpha1$ with an extra redundant copy of residues 12-70 (Figure 1A) giving a final 142 amino-acid residues (Mw 16. 5 kDa). It is "trivalent" with one extra free –SH group (Cys-15) that is able to interact with an additional $\alpha\beta$ unit. As such, one $\alpha2\beta$ unit binds to either $\alpha1\beta$ or $\alpha2\beta$ to form large polymers [($\alpha1\beta$)2-($\alpha2\beta$)n in Hp 2-1 and ($\alpha2\beta$)n in Hp 2-2] as shown in Figure 1B. Therefore, the different number of -SH sites produced from the two alleles lead to three phenotypes, each with a unique arrangement of polymers. For Hp 2-1, the ($\alpha2\beta$) units form linear polymer chains, elongating until two ($\alpha1\beta$) units bind to each side of ($\alpha2\beta$)n so that ($\alpha1\beta$)($\alpha2\beta$)n($\alpha1\beta$) polymers are formed. Notably, these polymers contain Hp 1-1 molecules, but not 2-2. For Hp 2-2 lacking of($\alpha1\beta$), the basic ($\alpha2\beta$) units initially form linear polymers until the two endslink together to form a cyclic complex ($\alpha2\beta$)n as illustrated in Figure 1B. These types of polymer structure have been confirmed by electron microscopic images [7].

Hp binds Hb with an extremely high affinity [2] and the latter possessing an endogenous peroxidase activity, it becomes a simple and popular routine method to identify the Hp phenotype using a peroxidase based colorimetric-substrate [8, 9]. As shown in Figure 1C, it is rather convenient to distinguish the phenotypes Hp 2-1 and 2-2 by observing the presence of ($\alpha1\beta$)2 dimers and ($\alpha1\beta$)2($\alpha2\beta$) trimers in Hp 2-1 and the presence of other higher order polymers in Hp 2-2. Interestingly, we have found that there are only few cyclic trimers among the Hp 2-2 polymers as compared to that of large intermediate polymers (Figure 1C). The variance in polymeric forms of Hp 2-1 and 2-2 and the mechanism by which Hp 2-1 possesses ($\alpha1\beta$)2 with no cyclic ($\alpha2\beta$)n have not been fully elucidated.

Clinically, the polymeric Hp phenotypes have been reported to be associated with the risk of kidney failure, diabetes, autoimmune, and cardiovascular diseases [6, 8, 10, 11].It is of interest to note that the plasma concentrations of Hp 1-1are found to be differentially higher than that of 2-1 and 2-2[8, 12]with values of 184 ±42, 153 ±55 or 93 ±54 mg/dL for Hp 1-1, 2-1 or 2-2, respectively [8].

The purpose of this study was to identify the possible number of polymers in each isolated Hp phenotypes 2-1 and 2-2 and to provide a theory for the Hp polymer assembly from our experimental data. We hypothesized that steric hindrance acts as a limiting factor on the formation of Hp 2-2 trimers. Finally, we addressed the differentially higher plasma levels of Hp 1-1 than 2-1 and 2-2 in normal subjects based on mRNA levels. A predominant gene activity of *Hp 1* greater than *Hp 2* was proposed.

2. Number of polymers in Hp phenotypes

To determine the number of polymeric forms of Hp 1-1, 2-1, and 2-2, plasma Hp isolated from a monoclonal antibody affinity-column [13]was first analyzed on a SDS-PAGE. A typical example showing the polymer numbers of Hp 2-2 is depicted in Figure 3. Western blot analysis confirms that each band actually corresponds to each size of the Hp polymer using a monoclonal antibody specific to the Hp α-chain (Figure 3B). Similar to that previously described [14, 15], the resolution using SDS-PAGE was not quite satisfactory. We then utilized a native-PAGE that gave a better resolution of higher polymers. Figure 3 shows that Hp 1-1 possesses a single homogenous form or ($\alpha\beta$)2 as expected, while Hp 2-1 or 2-2 possesses ($\alpha\beta$)2, trimer, tetramer, pentamer, and other polymers consistent to those depicted in Figure 2. The visible number of Hp 2-1 polymers is approximately up to 9 or ($\alpha\beta$)10, starting with ($\alpha1\beta$)2. Remarkably interesting, there are as many as 18 polymers or ($\alpha\beta$)20 seen in Hp 2-2, which have not been previously identified in terms of the polymeric number.

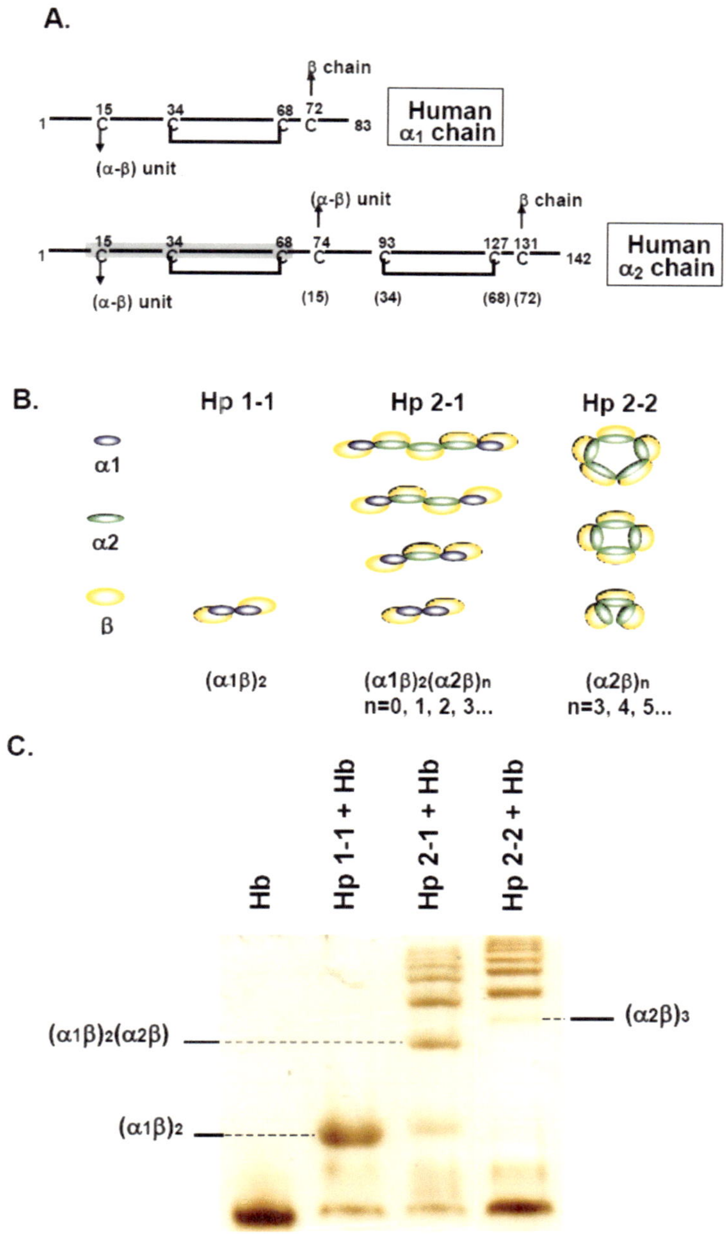

Figure 1. Polymeric structures of Hp 1-1, 2-1 and 2-2. Haptoglobin polymers are made up of (αβ) units with different number of –thiol groups in α1β and α2β. A) Schematic view of α1 and α2 chains encoded by the *Hp 1* and *Hp 2* alleles, respectively. The –COOH terminal Cys-72 of α1 always links to a β chain forming αβ basic unit. Whereas α2 contains a tandem repeat of residues 12-70 with Cys-15 and -74 linking to other αβ units, making the α2"trivalent". B) Illustrative view of the arrangement of (αβ) unit in each Hp phenotype, where n represents the repeat unit. C) 7% Native-PAGE of Hp-hemoglobin complexes showing the characteristics of polymeric pattern of each phenotype. Such complexes are used for Hp phenotyping. Of note, the amount of cyclic Hp 2-2 trimer or (α2β)3 is relatively limited.

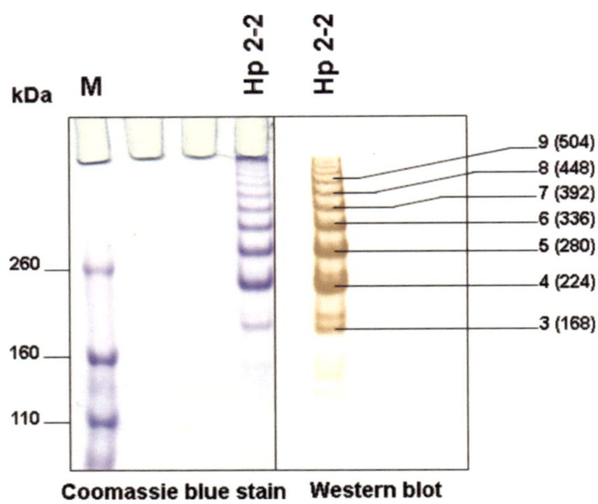

Figure 2. SDS–PAGE of isolated human Hp 2-2. Molecular patterns of polymeric Hp 2-2 using 4% non-reducing SDS—PAGE, showing the heterogeneous nature (left). The identity of each polymeric band is further confirmed by Western blot analysis using a α chain specific mAb (W1) prepared against Human Hp(right).

3. Decreasing concentration of Hp polymers determine the higher polymer numbers of Hp 2-2 than that of Hp 2-1

In addition to the number of Hp polymers, it is of interest to note that the concentration of each polymer is almost conversely correlated to the number of repeated (αβ) units. To substantiate the above observation, the relative intensity of each polymer within the Hp 2-1 or 2-2 was determined using an image analysis. Figure 4 demonstrates that the concentration of each polymer (except from Hp 2-1 dimer and Hp 2-2 trimer, discussed below) gradually decreases when the number of repeated units increases. The regression of arbitrary polymer concentration is found to be exponentially dependent on the number of repeated (αβ) units (starting from the trimer for Hp 2-1 and tetramer for Hp 2-2) leading to anequation for Hp 2-1 as:

$$\left[\mathrm{Pn}\right] = 6.4929{*}e^{-0.5286n} \qquad (1)$$

Where, n (≥ 3) represents the number of repeated units. [Pn] is the arbitrary protein concentration at the denoted number of repeated (αβ) units (n). The concentration of large polymers eventually attenuates to zero as the polymer number increases. Similarly, the equation for Hp 2-2 is:

http://dx.doi.org/10.5772/56048

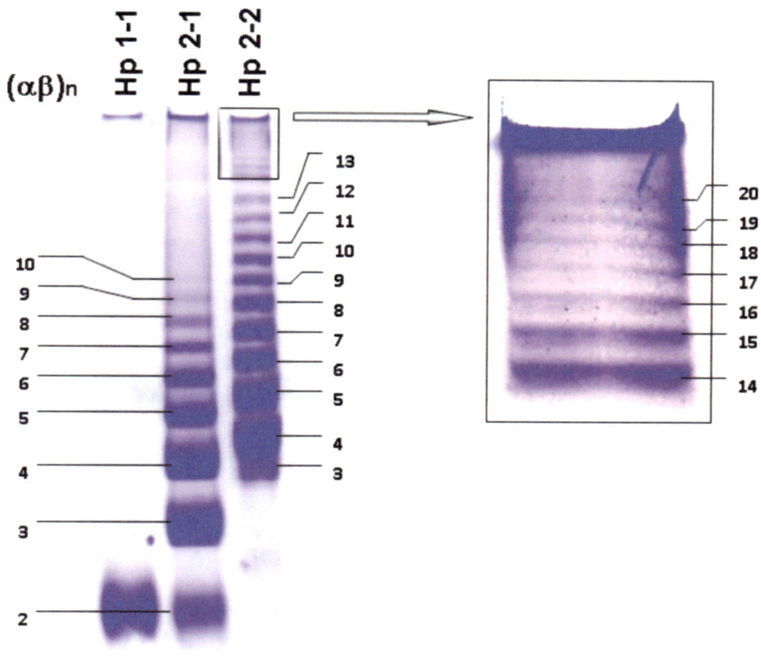

Figure 3. Native-PAGE of isolated human Hp 1-1, 2-1 and 2-2. For Hp 1-1 there is only a single homodimer or (α1β)2 observed, while polymers with as many as 10 and 20 repeated units can be seen in Hp 2-1 and Hp 2-2, respectively.

$$\left[Pn\right] = 3.1783^{*}e^{-0.3319n} \tag{2}$$

Where $n \geq 4$

An exponential decrease is recognized as the solution to the differential equation:

$$\frac{d[p]}{dn} = -k\left[p\right] \tag{3}$$

This means that the relationship (or ratio) between the concentration of polymers at number n+1 and n is constant. For Hp 2-1, the quotient derived form Eq. (1) is:

$$6.4929^{*}e^{-0.5286\,(n+1)} / \, 6.4929^{*}e^{-0.5286\,n} = 0.59 \tag{4}$$

For Hp 2-2, the quotient from Eq. (2) is:

$$3.1783 * e^{-0.3319\,(n+1)} \,/\, 3.1783 * e^{-0.3319n} = 0.72 \qquad (5)$$

Of notice that at a given protein concentration of Hp, the total number of detectable polymers for Hp 2-1 would be significantly less than that of 2-2. This is because the quotient in Eq. (4) is smaller, the protein concentration [Pn] approaches to zero faster (as n increases) when compared to Eq. (5).

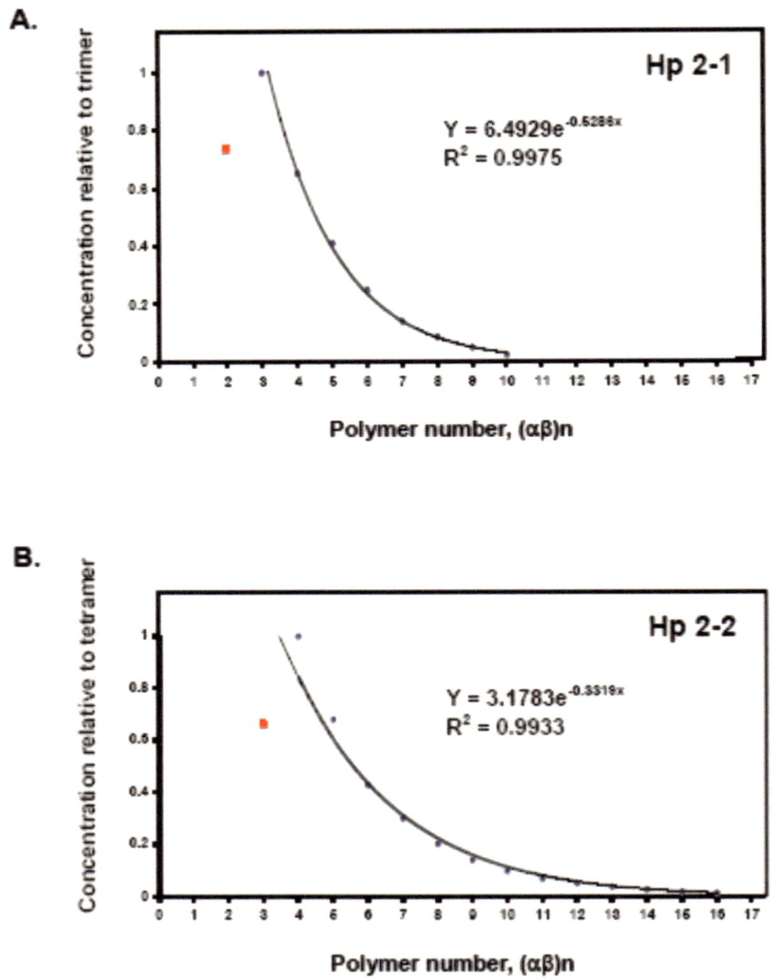

Figure 4. Plot of the polymer concentration as a function of (αβ)repeated number. A) Each polymer concentration of Hp 2-1 derived from Figure 3 is presented with the relative ratio to Hp trimer. The dimer is excluded from the exponential regression line since its concentration is beyond or below that proposed mathematical model (see text). B) Similarly, the trimer is excluded from the regression line as described above.

http://dx.doi.org/10.5772/56048

4. Possible kinetics for the assembly of Hp polymers

As shown in Figure 4 and Eq. (1) and (2), the concentration of the denoted polymer decreases exponentially with increasing polymer number. One of the attractive modes of elongation in polymer assembly (based on the exponential decrease in concentration) is that the polymer can be constructed by the addition of one (αβ)-unit at a time. This model assumes that reactions between already existing polymers are ignored. For example, a reaction such as: (α2β)n+1 and (α2β)n-1 to form (α2β)2n is not considered. However, if the reactions are multiples as that depicted in Figure 5, the possible assembly pathways of a given tetramer or hexamer would be complicated. Under the latter circumstance (Figure 5), once these multiple reactions take place it would generate a given polymer at different rates. We cannot rule out this possibility at the present time. The addition of one (αβ)-unit at a time is a simple model that gives rise to an exponential decrease with quotient remaining to be constant when applied to the number of polymers formed in each Hp phenotype. Despite the feasibility of the "one at a time" model, the overall rate of formation of polymers would be:

$$R_n > R_{n+1} \quad (6)$$

Where R_n is the formation rate of a denoted polymer with n repeated units, starting with n = 3 for Hp 2-1 and n = 4 for Hp 2-2 (Figure 4) (discussed below). It means that the smaller the polymers, the higher rate of assembly.

5. Proposed scheme for the formation of Hp 2-1 linear polymers

It has been well established that Hp 2-1 polymers, attributed by heterozygous *Hp 1* and *Hp 2*, are in a linear form (Figure 1). One essential question we attempted to address is why an Hp1-1 molecule can be seen without cyclic Hp 2-2 polymers in Hp 2-1 populations (Figures. 1 and 3). As depicted in Figure 6A, the gene responsible for the synthesis of α1β and α2β are from the *Hp 1* and *Hp 2* alleles, respectively. In theory, some α2β should be able to form 2-2 cyclic polymers. We speculated that the overall α1β-mRNA synthesized might be greater than the α2β-mRNA, which is in favor of the initial assembly of Hp 1-1 dimer (α1β)2. To test this hypothesis, we used the HepG2 cell line which by coincidence belongs to the Hp 2-1 genotype. We then determined the expression levels of the *Hp 1* and *Hp 2* alleles over time using RT-PCR, while utilizing LDL as an acute phase stimulant [8]. Figure 6B and C demonstrate that the expression of the *Hp 1* allele is significantly superior to *Hp 2* through all the induction times. In a previous study, we also reported that the synthesis rate of α1β was significantly faster than that of α2β after induction [8].

First, we proposed that the excessive (α1β) units naturally self-assemble into Hp 1-1 molecules. Second, because each (α2β)-unit contains two -SH open ends, (α2β) units must initially self-assemble into (α2β)n regardless of the presence of (α1β), where n ≥ 2. As shown in Figure 7 using a pentamer as an example, the reaction of cyclization of (α2β)n may take a long time in

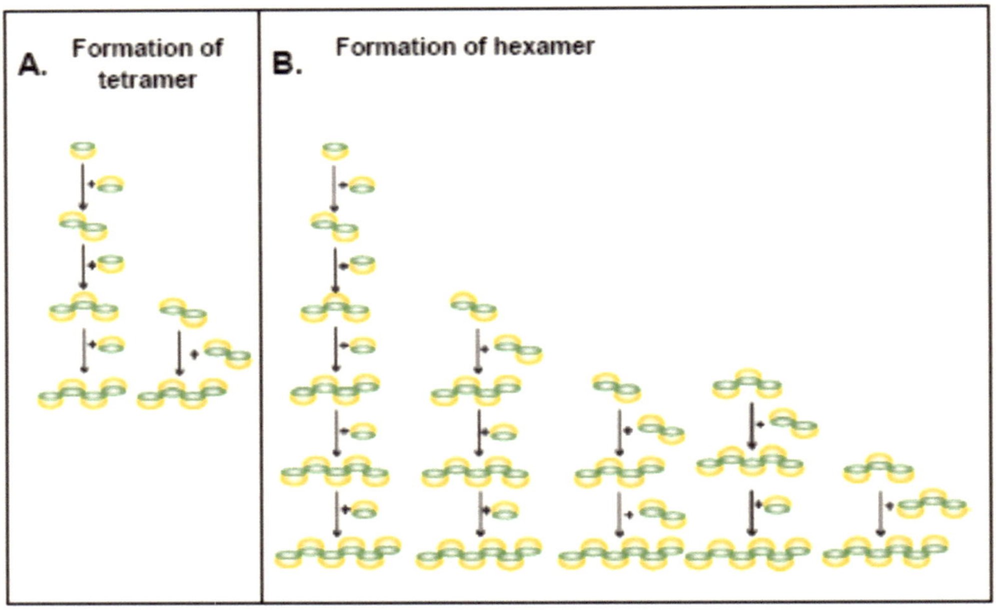

Figure 5. Schematic view of large and small polymers assembled through multiple reaction pathways. A) An example using tetramer as a model for two pathway assembling, one is by adding one unit at a time and the other is via a reaction between the two dimers. B) An example using hexamer as a model to illustrate there are five possible pathways, including by adding one unit at a time and by reactions between already formed polymers.

the process of polymer refolding. The rate of cyclization in theory is slower than the formation of linear polymers. In the presence of excess (α1β) units, these (α2β)5 polymers in linear form could be terminated by the addition of (α1β) at both ends. The resulting product is, therefore, in a linear form.

Furthermore, Figure 8 shows that one (α1β) and one (α2β) can also form (α1β)-(α2β)-, but is terminated with an addition of a (α1β) which gives rise to the smallest heterogeneous linear polymer (α1β)-(α2β)-(α1β). However, if the next addition is a (α2β), then further extension by coupling an (α1β)- or (α2β)-unit is possible. Thus, the next linear polymer is a tetramer or (α1β)-(α2β)-(α2β)-(α1β), otherwise the elongation continues until the addition of a (α1β). If the portion of open-end polymers (α1β) (α2β)n- that adds (α2β) or (α1β) is independent of the number of repeated (αβ)-units (n) within the polymers, then the relationship between the rate of addition of (α1β) and (α2β) does not change. Thus, the concentration of polymers depending on size would follow an approximately exponential decrease since a constant portion of an open end polymers adds (α1β) and a constant portion adds (α2β) (Figure 8). However, since there are two different pathways leading to polymers with only one open end (Figure 7), the decrease is truly exponential if the (α1β) are added in same positions for the both pathways.

Explaining the low abundance of dimers or (α1β)2 in Hp 2-1of Figure 3 is somewhat difficult. One possible explanation is that formation of the (α1β)2 is terminated and limited by the presence of (α2β)-subunits. If this was the case, the reactivity of the (α2β) could be higher than

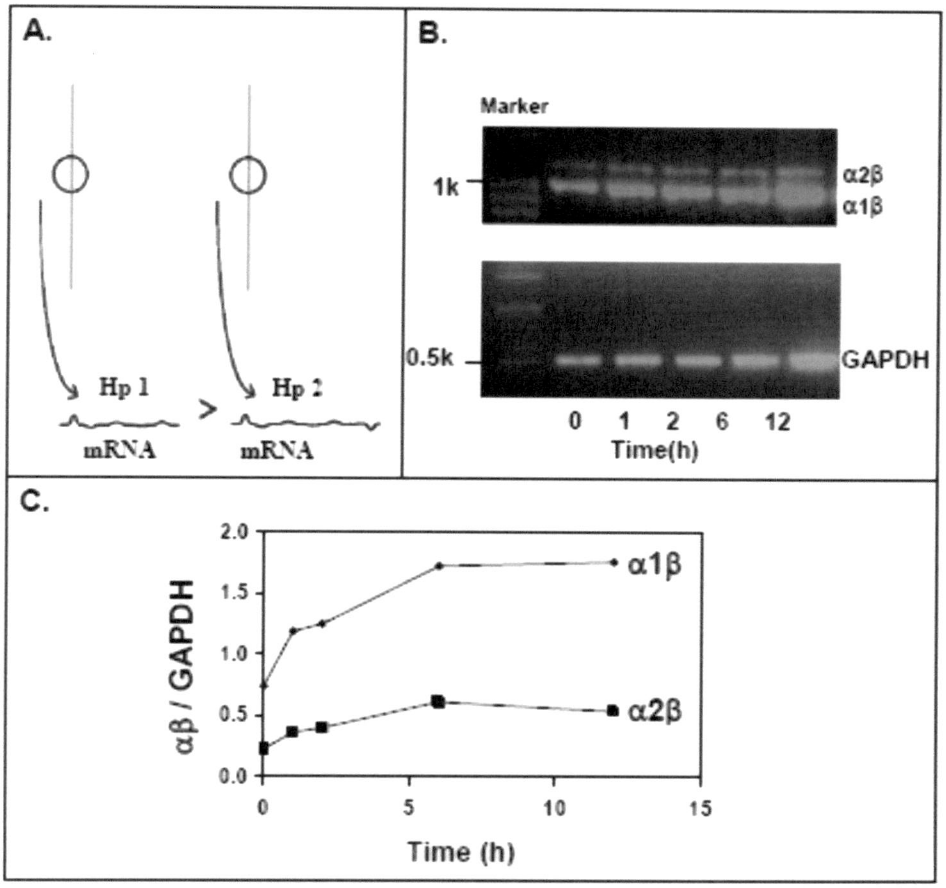

Figure 6. Schematic view of the molecular expression of α1β and α2β unit and its level induced by LDL. A) *Hp 1* and *Hp 2* alleles are responsible for making the mRNA of α1β and α2β polypeptides, respectively. B) RT-PCR showing the overall synthesis of α1β is greater than α2β m-RNA over time, while the house keeping gene GAPDH was used as a control. C) The intensity of the α1β band is higher than that of α2β at all induction times as determined using an image analysis.

that of (α1β) in terms of the binding to the other (αβ)-units. Nevertheless, it is a fact that the concentration of Hp 1-1 determined in Hp 2-1 polymers is not fit into the exponential decrement curve shown in Figure 4A.

6. Proposed scheme for the formation of Hp 2-2 cyclic polymers

As shown in Figure 9, each basic (α2β) unit initially forms linear polymers with both ends having one thiol group open for further subunit extension. The elongation terminated until the free ends bind together to form a cyclic Hp 2-2. According to Eq. (5), the quotient between

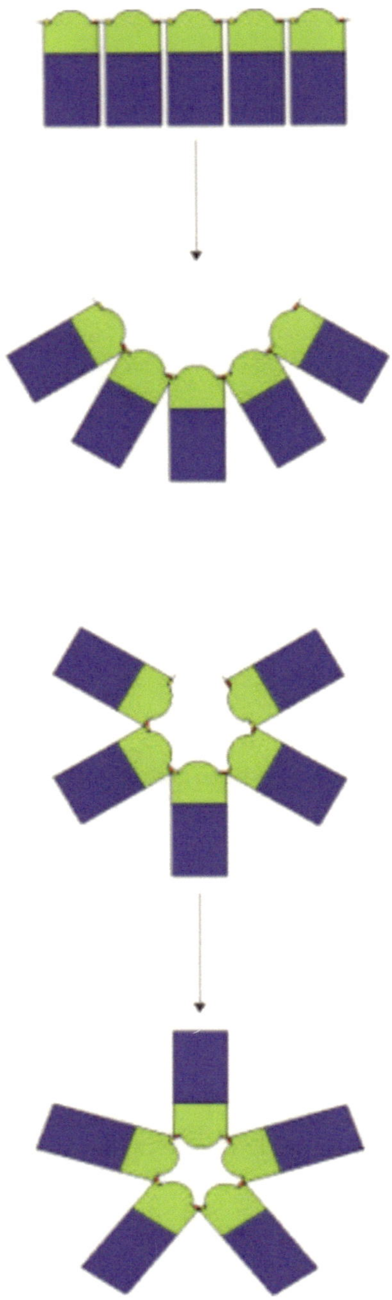

Figure 7. Model of cyclization of Hp polymers. Regardless of the pathways involved in the formation of (α2β)n, a given pentamer or (α2β)5 requires a correct conformation to be cyclized. The rate of the process is therefore slower than uncyclized form. The uncylized (α2β)n could be initially present in the polymer populations during the assembly of Hp 2-1 molecules. However in the presence of excess of basic (α1β) units, the remaining uncyclized forms are terminated by coupling a (α1β). If (α2β) units are in excess, the cyclization of Hp 2-2 polymers should be allowed in theory.

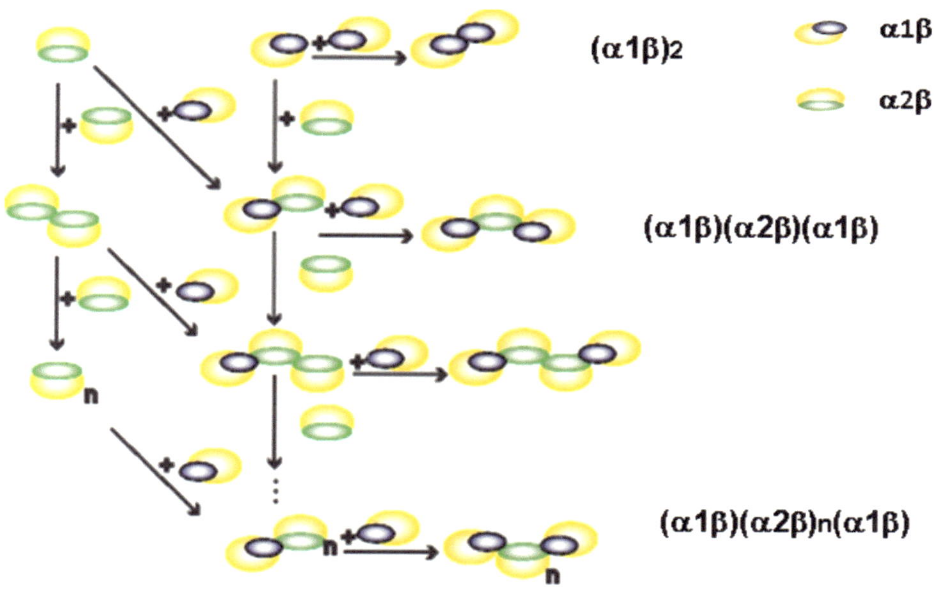

Figure 8. Proposed model for the format on of Hp 2-1 linear polymers. Nucleation occurs through the reaction between the two αβ units with the possible products: a simple (α1β)2 dimer is initially formed without further extension because of the saturation of free -thiol groups. The next linear trimer is formed with the addition of two (α1β) units to one (α2β). Notably, either (α1β) or (α2β) may subsequently add to one (α2β) unit until both ends are bound with (α1β).

polymers of order n+1 and n is 0. 72. It means that 72% of the polymers with free –SH would link another (α2β) to form the next higher order polymer. It equals to:

$$\text{Rate of addition } \alpha 2\beta \ / \ (\text{Rate addition of } \alpha 2\beta + \text{Rate of cyclic formation}) = 0.72. \tag{7}$$

Which equals to:

$$\text{Rate of cyclic formation} = 0.39 \ * \text{rate of addition of } \alpha 2\beta. \tag{8}$$

It is seen from Eqs. (7) and (8) that the formation of a cyclic polymer is slow as compared to the addition of a (α2β)unit. In other words the ratio between the next order of a polymer and a given polymer remains constant or 72% (Figure 3). This is thought to be the reason for the large polymer numbers seen in the Hp 2-2 phenotype. The slow rate of cyclic formation further explains why there are no cyclic (α2β)n polymers found in the Hp 2-1 population. However, if the overall synthesis of (α2β) molecules was in excess in the individuals possessing both *Hp 1* and *Hp* heterozygote (Hp 2-1 phenotype), we would see the cyclic polymers regardless of the slow rate involved in the cyclization. Nevertheless, the rate of cyclization derived here is consistent to that we proposed in Figure 7.

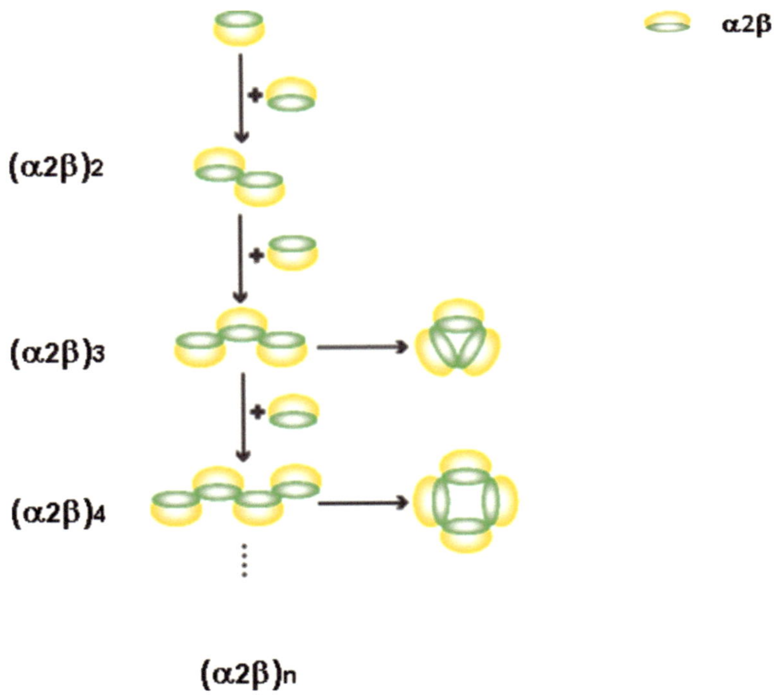

Figure 9. Hypothetical model for the formation of cyclic polymers. Nucleation occurs through the reaction between two (α2β) in creating a first linear (α2β)2. Formation of a stacked dimer is not possible due to the steric hindrance between the two -thiol groups of each subunit (deoicted in Figure 10). As such it initially forms a linear trimer or (α2β)3 prior to the cyclization. This linear trimer can then either be elongated by the addition of other (α2β)n, or otherwise be terminated by a subsequent cyclization.

7. Steric hindrance could explain the low abundance of trimer in Hp 2-2 phenotype

A fascinating phenomena is that the concentration of Hp 2-2 trimers or (α2β)3 seen in Hp-Hb complex is extremely low in human plasma of all the Hp 2-2 subjects that we have investigated without exception (Figure 1C). Its concentration does not fit the mathematical model (Figure 3 and eq. 2). As depicted in Figure 10, we hypothesized that there is a steric hindrance between the two free thiol groups of a (α2β) unit. First, under this condition the hindrance totally abolishes the formation of a basic dimer (α2β)2. Second, steric hindrance prevents the cross-linking from forming a trimer to some extent due to limited space in the central space. This may account for the low abundance of trimers in Hp 2-2 polymers. Third, as the central space increases, the hindrance does not substantially affect the formation of a tetramer, a pentamer, or larger polymers. Recently, we also demostrated an unique tetrameric structure of deer plasma Hp which cna explain an evolutionary advantage in the Hp 2-2 phenotype with homogeneous structure[16].

http://dx.doi.org/10.5772/56048

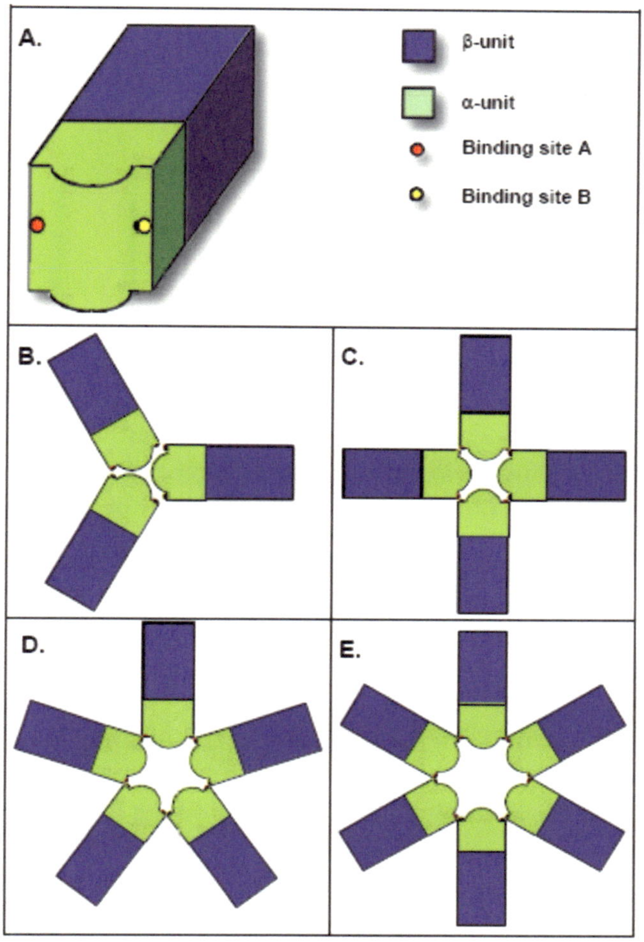

Figure 10. Proposed model of the assembling of Hp 2-2 polymers with limited trimer molecules. A) The two -thiol groups linking the Hp subunits into polymers are located at a plane where they are separated by a steric hindrance. Under this condition the hindrance prevents the formation of a basic dimer (α2β)2. B) The trimer is able to form to some extent, but is limited by the hindrance that accounts for its low abundance. C-E) The polymers of order four and higher are assembled without any steric hindrance as the central space getting wider.

8. Plasma Hp 1-1 levels are differentially greater than Hp 2-1 and 2-2

It has been known that plasma levels of Hp 1-1 are dramatically higher than 2-1 and 2-2 in normal human subjects. Order of the levels is Hp 1-1 > Hp 2-1 > Hp 2-2 with plasma concentrations of about 180, 150 and 90 mg/dL, respectively [8]. The mechanism involved in such discrepancy, however, has not been explored. As shown in Figure 6A, there are two alleles *Hp 1* and *Hp 2* responsible for the specific synthesis of the ($\alpha 1\beta$) and ($\alpha 2\beta$) subunits, respectively. Based on the RT-PCR analysis of allele expression using a HepG2 cell line containing both alleles, it appears that the amount of mRNA produced by the *Hp 1* allele is significantly greater than that of *Hp 2* over time (Figure 6B-C). Thus, it explains why the plasma concentration of Hp in subjects with *Hp 1* is markedly higher than that with *Hp 2-1*(heterozygote) or *Hp 2*(homozygote). Although the reason for low expression of the *Hp 2* allele remains unclear, we proposed that the gene activity of *Hp 1* is superior to *Hp 2*.

9. Clinical significance of Hp phenotypes

The Hp is an acute-phase protein in response to infection and inflammation. It is also one of the most abundant serum proteins with high potency of anti inflammation and antioxidant activities [17, 18];therefore render its availability for maintaining homeostasis. Anyaberrancein expression levels or subfraction composition of Hp may possibly be used to establish valuable diagnostic or prognostic indicator in various diseases. Human Hp polymorphism is not only determined by unique genetic duplication, but also affected by complex assembly processes.

Reports regarding the relationship between the plasma levels and diseases remain rare owing to the difficulty and complexicity in precised determination of Hp levels in different individuals with different phenotypes. We have shown for the first time that immunoassay (such as ELISA) for Hp measurement has to use Hp phenotype-matched standard for one individual with one specific phenotype (ie., one Hp 1-1 subject needs Hp 1-1 protein as a standard used for calibration) due to the different biochemical structure and immunochemical properties among the Hp phenotypes. Following this concept, we have established an accurate ELISA test for measurement of Hp levels [8]. Clinically, we discovered that the patients with normal acute-phase response in Hp elevation in sepsis had fewer events of multiple-organ dysfunction and lower mortality rate. The Hp2-2 phenotype is associated with failure to increase plasma Hp levels in the acute stage of sepsis (unpublished data). In another study, we showed that one short-term jogging and explosive run are able to induce a substantial elevation of Hp in peripheral blood. In mice, Hp levels are elevated significantly and concomitantly with the increase in neutrophils over the circulation following a 2-week exercise [19]. This finding not only suggests that acute net increase in Hp levels may be directly derived from the neutrophils but also indicates that Hp could be a biomarker for the neutrophil functional activity.

It is well known thatcardiovascular eventsin diabetic patients are closely linked to the Hp2-2 phenotype [20]. Recently, accumulating evidence showed that Hp elevation implies various biologic meaning. Notably, elevated Hp concentrations in cord blood of newborns have been identified as a biomarker to predict the occurrence of early-onset neonatal sepsis [21-23]. In patients with chronic inflammatory demyelinating polyneuropathy (CIDP) and multiple sclerosis,Hp levels in cerebral spinal fluid are high [24]. Serum Hp is also a useful predictive biomarker for steroid therapy efficacy in the treatment of idiopathic nephrotic syndrome[25]. Plasma Hp concentrations are elevated in patients with abdominal aortic aneurysm, particularly those with the Hp 2-2 phenotype [26].

http://dx.doi.org/10.5772/56048

10. Conclusions

Regardless of the hypothetical model, the discovery of an exponential decrease in concentration between (αβ)n and (αβ)n+1 is of remarkable interest. It provides insight into the role of Hp polymer size involved in the clinical outcomes and physiological functions. The maximal number of repeated (αβ) units we reported here is as many as 10 for Hp 2-1 and 20 for 2-2. Should the concentration not follow an exponential decrement, the maximal number of polymers assembled could have been much larger. We suggest a simple kinetics model with the excessive synthesis of (α1β) units that can explain the lack of cyclic polymers in the Hp 2-1 individuals. We also proposed that the allele activity of *Hp 1* is superior to *Hp 2*, which accounts for the differentially greater Hp concentrations in Hp 1-1 human subjects than in Hp 2-1 and 2-2. Finally,we speculated that Hp polymorphism from genetic sequence and protein assembly may reflect the response to inflammation. The application of Hp in clinical medicine awaits further investigations.

Acknowledgements

This work was supported by National Science Council, Taiwan, ROC [NSC 95-2313-B-009-03-MY2 to SJM, 100-2314-B-010-001-MY2, and 100-2314-B-010-044-MY3 to CYC]; and National Yang Ming University Hospital, Ilan, Taiwan, ROC [RD2011-007, RD2012-006 and RD2013-005 to CYC]; and by The Friends of Chalmers scholarship foundation.

Author details

Mikael Larsson[1,2], Tsai-Mu Cheng[1,3], Cheng-Yu Chen[4,5,6] and Simon J. T. Mao[1]

*Address all correspondence to: doctormao888@gmail.com

1 Research Institute of Biochemical Engineering, Department of Biological Science and Technology, National Chiao Tung University, Hsinchu, Taiwan, ROC

2 Department of Chemical and Biological Engineering, Chalmers University of Technology, Gothenburg, Sweden

3 Taipei Medical University, Taipei, Taiwan, ROC

4 Department of Internal Medicine, Nation Yang-Ming University Hospital, Ilan, Taiwan, ROC

5 Institute of Clinical Medicine, National Yang-Ming University, Taipei, Taiwan, ROC

6 Cardinal Tien College of Healthcare and Management, Taipei. Taiwan, ROC

References

[1] Tseng CF, Lin CC, Huang HY, Liu HC, Mao SJ. Antioxidant role of human haptoglobin. Proteomics. 2004;4(8):2221-8.

[2] Wicher KB, Fries E. Haptoglobin, a hemoglobin-binding plasma protein, is present in bony fish and mammals but not in frog and chicken. Proceedings of the National Academy of Sciences of the United States of America. 2006;103(11):4168-73.

[3] Kristiansen M, Graversen JH, Jacobsen C, Sonne O, Hoffman HJ, Law SK, et al. Identification of the haemoglobin scavenger receptor. Nature. 2001;409(6817):198-201.

[4] Nielsen MJ, Petersen SV, Jacobsen C, Thirup S, Enghild JJ, Graversen JH, et al. A unique loop extension in the serine protease domain of haptoglobin is essential for CD163 recognition of the haptoglobin-hemoglobin complex. The Journal of biological chemistry. 2007;282(2):1072-9.

[5] Feng Tseng C, T. Mao SJ. Analysis of Antioxidant as a Therapeutic Agent for Atherosclerosis. Current Pharmaceutical Analysis. 2006;2(4):16.

[6] Langlois MR, Delanghe JR. Biological and clinical significance of haptoglobin polymorphism in humans. Clinical chemistry. 1996;42(10):1589-600.

[7] Wejman JC, Hovsepian D, Wall JS, Hainfeld JF, Greer J. Structure and assembly of haptoglobin polymers by electron microscopy. Journal of molecular biology. 1984;174(2):343-68.

[8] Cheng TM, Pan JP, Lai ST, Kao LP, Lin HH, Mao SJ. Immunochemical property of human haptoglobin phenotypes: determination of plasma haptoglobin using type-matched standards. Clinical biochemistry. 2007;40(13-14):1045-56.

[9] Delanghe J, Allcock K, Langlois M, Claeys L, De Buyzere M. Fast determination of haptoglobin phenotype and calculation of hemoglobin binding capacity using high pressure gel permeation chromatography. Clinica chimica acta; international journal of clinical chemistry. 2000;291(1):43-51.

[10] Levy AP. Application of pharmacogenomics in the prevention of diabetic cardiovascular disease: mechanistic basis and clinical evidence for utilization of the haptoglobin genotype in determining benefit from antioxidant therapy. Pharmacology & therapeutics. 2006;112(2):501-12.

[11] Nakhoul FM, Miller-Lotan R, Awaad H, Asleh R, Levy AP. Hypothesis--haptoglobin genotype and diabetic nephropathy. Nature clinical practice Nephrology. 2007;3(6): 339-44.

[12] Densem CG, Wassel J, Cooper A, Yonan N, Brooks NH, Keevil B. Haptoglobin phenotype correlates with development of cardiac transplant vasculopathy. The Journal

of heart and lung transplantation : the official publication of the International Society for Heart Transplantation. 2004;23(1):43-9.

[13] Tseng CF, Huang HY, Yang YT, Mao SJ. Purification of human haptoglobin 1-1, 2-1, and 2-2 using monoclonal antibody affinity chromatography. Protein expression and purification. 2004;33(2):265-73.

[14] Fuller GM, Rasco MA, McCombs ML, Barnett DR, Bowman BH. Subunit composition of haptoglobin 2-2 polymers. Biochemistry. 1973;12(2):253-8.

[15] Hooper DC, Peacock AC. Determination of the subunit composition of haptoglobin 2-1 polymers using quantitative densitometry of polyacrylamide gels. The Journal of biological chemistry. 1976;251(19):5845-51.

[16] Lai IH, Lin KY, Larsson M, Yang MC, Shiau CH, Liao MH, et al. A unique tetrameric structure of deer plasma haptoglobin--an evolutionary advantage in the Hp 2-2 phenotype with homogeneous structure. FEBS J. 2008;275(5):981-93.

[17] Roche CJ, Dantsker D, Alayash AI, Friedman JM. Enhanced nitrite reductase activity associated with the haptoglobin complexed hemoglobin dimer: functional and antioxidative implications. Nitric Oxide. 2012;27(1):32-9.

[18] Purushothaman KR, Purushothaman M, Levy AP, Lento PA, Evrard S, Kovacic JC, et al. Increased expression of oxidation-specific epitopes and apoptosis are associated with haptoglobin genotype: possible implications for plaque progression in human atherosclerosis. J Am Coll Cardiol. 2012;60(2):112-9.

[19] Chen CY, Hsieh WL, Lin PJ, Chen YL, Mao SJ. Haptoglobin is an Exercise-Responsive Acute-Phase Protein. Vienna: InTech. 2011:289-302.

[20] Sadrzadeh SM, Bozorgmehr J. Haptoglobin phenotypes in health and disorders. Am J Clin Pathol. 2004;121 Suppl:S97-104.

[21] Buhimschi CS, Bhandari V, Dulay AT, Nayeri UA, Abdel-Razeq SS, Pettker CM, et al. Proteomics mapping of cord blood identifies haptoglobin "switch-on" pattern as biomarker of early-onset neonatal sepsis in preterm newborns. PLoS One. 2011;6(10):e26111.

[22] Chavez-Bueno S, Beasley JA, Goldbeck JM, Bright BC, Morton DJ, Whitby PW, et al. 'Haptoglobin concentrations in preterm and term newborns'. J Perinatol. 2011;31(7): 500-3.

[23] Philip AG. Haptoglobin in diagnosis of sepsis. J Perinatol. 2012;32(4):312; author reply 3.

[24] Zhang HL, Zhang XM, Mao XJ, Deng H, Li HF, Press R, et al. Altered cerebrospinal fluid index of prealbumin, fibrinogen, and haptoglobin in patients with Guillain-Barre syndrome and chronic inflammatory demyelinating polyneuropathy. Acta Neurol Scand. 2012;125(2):129-35.

[25] Wen Q, Huang LT, Luo N, Wang YT, Li XY, Mao HP, et al. Proteomic Profiling Identifies Haptoglobin as a Potential Serum Biomarker for Steroid-Resistant Nephrotic Syndrome. Am J Nephrol. 2012;36(2):105-13.

[26] Pan JP, Cheng TM, Shih CC, Chiang SC, Chou SC, Mao SJ, et al. Haptoglobin phenotypes and plasma haptoglobin levels in patients with abdominal aortic aneurysm. J Vasc Surg. 2011;53(5):1189-94.